SET FREE

A Guide to Inner Healing and Deliverance

Steve Dominguez

Endorsements

"The greatest need at this hour of the Church's assignment to advance the Kingdom of God through bringing wholeness to the world is for the provision of practical, easy to understand, and activation tools to bring healing and freedom. *Set Free* by Steve Dominguez is that tool that will become a significant part of your ministry "toolbox" to enable you to walk in the confidence of your God-given authority and power. Steve brings years of experience to this and is a trustworthy source of God's revelation on this subject. I wholeheartedly endorse this equipping manual for your use."

Dr. Mike Hutchings
Director of Education, Global Awakening
President, God Heals PTSD Foundation

"The average American Christian is more like a civilian on vacation than a soldier at war. The average American Christian knows next to nothing about the armor of God, the spiritual weapons God has given us and how to use them, or our identity and authority as believers in Christ. Here is a very timely and helpful book that has the potential to equip many thousands of Christians to more effectively navigate in the spiritual realm and to walk in the authority and victory over the enemy that are ours in Jesus Christ. Steve Dominguez (my good friend and ministry partner) has a wealth of experience in setting captives free in Christ. His book is written in a very readable style and is filled with practical teaching, wisdom, ministry guidelines, and helpful suggestions. The many stories of miraculous deliverances and healings in people's lives are tremendously inspiring and faith-building. I heartily endorse this book and hope that you are as encouraged as I am after learning from its pages."

Dr. Clayton Ford, speaker, author, and
National Co-Director of Holy Spirit Renewal Ministries

"I am thrilled that Steve Dominguez has just released this life-changing book *Set Free.* This book is so practical and powerful and simplifies the process of getting free or helping others get free from demonic strongholds and staying free in Christ.

I have worked closely with Steve and his wonderful wife Risa for several years now. They are part of our core leadership team at Love Says Go Ministries International. I have recognized that Steve and Risa have a powerful calling on their lives to set the captives free and to train others in this most important ministry.

Through the years, I have watched Steve and Risa bring freedom to many through Christ's redemption for physical healing, deliverance from the demonic, and inner healing. They walk in great Godly humility, character, authority and power. I recommend Steve and Risa personally to the highest level and their calling to train the body of Christ in freedom.

Set Free is an incredible book to help bring you into freedom or help you bring others into freedom. Maybe you or someone you know is struggling to stop feeling hopeless about something or a situation or maybe can't seem to stay free from an addictive behavior...this book is for you! *Set Free* has the tools and the empowerment from the Holy Spirit to really bring lasting freedom into believers' lives.

I love that Steve combines truth from God's word, powerful testimonies, practical action steps and prayers to partner with God's power to activate and maintain freedom into our lives. I do not think I have seen an easier, step by step guide to powerfully bring others into freedom like Steve has put together in *Set Free.* Whether you are looking for more freedom for yourself or you want to be more equipped to help others get free this book is for you. I think *Set Free* should be on the shelf in every believer's home as a "how-to" book when dealing with the demonic and helping others with the powerful ministry of setting the captives free!"

Jason Chin
Founder of Love Says Go Ministries International

Acknowledgements

I want to thank my wife, Risa, who has been an amazing partner in life and ministry. I couldn't imagine doing freedom sessions without her. Risa has been a great encouragement both in words and action. She has been a huge help in this area of ministry, second only to God and the host of heaven.

TABLE OF CONTENTS

INTRODUCTION

We are in a war. This was never more apparent to me than when I went with a small team to minster in India. Two brothers and a sister got in my line for ministry at a youth conference we were holding. The brothers were injured, and they were all sleeping outside of their house for fear of their lives. The reason for their fear was that the demonic threw them, or influenced them to jump, from two stories high. They said the night before that happened, a neighbor died. The night before their neighbor died, the house next to their neighbor's house had someone die. This was a daily pattern for about 5 nights in a row. I asked when this all started, and it turned out to be the day we left Chicago to go to India. The demonic tried to take them out before they could hear the gospel. Apparently, the demonic preferred to destroy rather than take a chance of losing possession. The three siblings had just received their new life in Christ that morning, but the brothers were still being tormented in their mind. Thankfully, I was able to set them free and bring healing to their wounds by the power of the Holy Spirit.

Jesus is the hope of the world. We need to preach it and demonstrate it. The intent of this book is to provide Biblically based assistance to a Christian desiring to help themselves or others walk in spiritual victory and freedom from demonic oppression.

I never set out in pursuit of this ministry. It sort of pursued me. My wife, Risa, and I started doing the ministry of physical healing years ago. It started to become apparent fairly quickly that not everything that appeared to be a physical aliment was always only physical. Many times there was a spirit behind the physical problem, creating it and resisting healing of it. And in some cases it was just a spirit of infirmity that needed to be removed.

Learning how to deal with these spirits to bring physical healing led to learning how to bring spiritual healing of emotions and mind as well. That eventually led to learning how to do more major deliverance of demonic oppression of all kinds.

The content of this book comes from years of learning by researching this subject, but most of all, hands on experience to learn what works best for what situation. Christians have access to a lot of spiritual weapons. There are different weapons to be used for different situations, just as with physical warfare. There are also different tactics and methods that can be used, but it's not about following a formula.

That being said, not only are there a lot of different situations that bring a need for spiritual freedom, there is a large degree of magnitude of demonization (the extent to which one is demonized) that can be on a person.

The term inner healing can mean different things to different people. One common definition is spiritual healing of emotions and mindsets. That is the definition that I would give, along with the clarification that while at times the affliction to be healed can produce very severe results, it doesn't have blatant manifestations such as demonic control of speech, change in image through contortion of face, or involuntary physical movement. The process of getting free from the latter is what I would define as deliverance ministry. However, to be clear, it's all a form of demonization or demonic oppression. This is why in all cases, my wife and I call our sessions freedom sessions. The goal is always the same: freedom from demonic oppression, control, torment, and influence.

The freedom sessions that my wife and I hold are not counseling sessions. While there may be a need to address a lifestyle issue, we are not counselors or life coaches. While I have nothing against counseling, our goal is always to get a person free of the demonic oppression and influence, no matter how severe, in one single session. We then provide the education to allow them to stay free on their own by teaching them about their identity and weapons of warfare. The goal is that those set free can walk out their freedom on their own.

GOD'S DESIRE FOR YOU TO BE SET FREE

In John chapter 2 we see Jesus, in what may seem to some as almost being out of character, as he takes a whip and drives those doing business out of the temple. In John 2:17 reference is made to Jesus' zeal which was prophesied in Psalm 69.

> Psalm 69:9
> Because zeal for Your house has eaten me up,
> And the reproaches of those who reproach You have fallen on me.

If Jesus, who is the perfect image of the Father (Hebrews 1:3), is that zealous to cleanse **that** temple, how much more will He be zealous to cleanse our bodies which now are temples of the Holy Spirit (1 Corinthians 6:19)? God is zealous for His own, and He will be quick to come to our rescue from the thief who comes to kill, steal, and destroy.

Setting free those in bondage was God's heart from the beginning.

Isaiah 61:1
The Spirit of the Lord God is upon Me,
Because the Lord has anointed Me
To preach good tidings to the poor;
He has sent Me to heal the brokenhearted,
To proclaim liberty to the captives,
And the opening of the prison to those who are bound;

Note a few things in this prophetic verse:
- The Lord's anointing –> the anointing of the Holy Spirit equips one for deliverance ministry
- To preach (or bring) good news (the gospel of the Kingdom) to the afflicted
- Healing the broken hearted (healing soul wounds)
- Liberty to the captives (captured by the enemy)
- Freedom to the prisoners (in bondage due to poor actions and choices)

In Luke 4 we see Jesus read this passage, and in Luke 4:23 He says, "Today this scripture is **fulfilled** in your hearing."

This prophesy was fulfilled with Jesus' ministry, which began with His anointing at His baptism. The power of the Holy Spirit is important to any ministry, and deliverance is no exception.

Jesus never stopped being the Son of God. Since authority is based on position and identity, Jesus still had the authority of the Son of God. However, He did come as a man, so He gave up His divine power. All the miracles He did were by the power of the Holy Spirit that came on Him for His ministry. This included casting out demons. This is why when accused of casting out demons by Beelzebub He warned them of blasphemy against the Holy Spirit.

Matthew 12:24-32

24 Now when the Pharisees heard it they said, "This fellow does not cast out demons except by Beelzebub, the ruler of the demons."

25 But Jesus knew their thoughts, and said to them: "Every kingdom divided against itself is brought to desolation, and every city or house divided against itself will not stand. 26 If Satan casts out Satan, he is divided against himself. How then will his kingdom stand? 27 And if I cast out demons by Beelzebub, by whom do your sons cast them out? Therefore, they shall be your judges. 28 But if I cast out demons by the Spirit of God, surely the kingdom of God has come upon you. 29 Or how can one enter a strong man's house and plunder his goods, unless he first binds the strong man? And then he will plunder his house. 30 He who is not with Me is against Me, and he who does not gather with Me scatters abroad.

31 Therefore I say to you, every sin and blasphemy will be forgiven men, but the blasphemy against the Spirit will not be forgiven men. 32 Anyone who speaks a word against the Son of Man, it will be forgiven him; but whoever speaks against the Holy Spirit, it will not be forgiven him, either in this age or in the age to come."

Later He passes this ministry to His disciples, and ultimately to His church.

Matthew 10:1

And when He had called His twelve disciples to Him, He gave them power over unclean spirits, to cast them out, and to heal all kinds of sickness and all kinds of disease.

He gave them power – or in other words, He delegated power (or authority to use power) to them.

The New International Version states is as follows.

Matthew 10:1 New International Version (NIV)
Jesus called his twelve disciples to him and gave them authority to drive out impure spirits and to heal every disease and sickness.

Mark 3:14-15
14 Then He appointed twelve, that they might be with Him and that He might send them out to preach, 15 and to have power to heal sicknesses and to cast out demons.

The word power in Mark 3:15 is *exousia* which means delegated authority. Exousia is the right to use *dunamis* (another word for power). Dunamis is the word used describing the power received when the Holy Spirit comes on you in Act 1:8 for ministry.

Exousia was power which was given to the disciples for ministry before Jesus went to the cross, and before the Holy Spirt had come upon the disciples.

Again, this is part of the Christian life. It's part of the great commission given in Mark.

Mark 16:17-18
17 And these signs will follow those who believe: In My name they will **cast out demons**; they will speak with new tongues; 18 they will **take up serpents**; and if they drink anything deadly, it will by no means hurt them; they will lay hands on the sick, and they will recover."

In verse 18 it says that they will take up serpents. Serpents are symbolic of the demonic. The Greek word used for take up is *airo*, which could also be translated "remove or take away." That gives a little more clarity to the verse.

Since setting people free from demonic oppression and bondage is part of the great commission as stated in the verses in Mark above, it should be a ministry made available at each church. The cross made it possible for healing to come to both our bodies and our souls. God's heart is health for both, but it's not automatic. Just as we pray for people to be physically healed, we need to apply what was made available through the cross for healing to the soul as well.

THE STEPS TO FREEDOM AND A NEW IDENTITY

Like the cliché', the first step to freedom is admitting there is a problem. Beyond that though, the person needing freedom needs to want to be free. Otherwise, it's just a waste of time for all involved. We've had parents bring teenagers to our house against their will. We, unfortunately, have to tell the parents we are not going to have a freedom session with their child if he or she doesn't want one. If they do want freedom, which is usually the case, we start with salvation, or recommitment to Christ if they are saved, and then proceed to apply all that Jesus made available through His death and resurrection.

Jesus dying on the cross is a giant legal action of God's grace allowing for all to be justified and set free from all spiritual bondage by taking steps of faith to receive the benefits of the sacrifice made on our behalf. However, when a person decides to receive the awesome gift of salvation offered by God through the sacrifice of His son Jesus as a propitiation for our sins, not all of the other benefits of Jesus' shed blood are automatically received. There are many other benefits made available that will once again need to be received by faith with declarations. Jesus didn't just die so that we could someday be in heaven. His actions took care of all aspects of sin, including shame,

9

guilt, torment, and ultimately death. Jesus made provision for the transformation of your spirit, and also for the healing of your body and soul. When a person gets saved, their spirit immediately gets redeemed and transformed. This is not true of the body and soul, but in the meantime we can experience healing and deliverance of sickness, disease, and torment. In the context of deliverance, the cross allows for freedom from demonic oppression, but it needs to be applied.

When Jesus raised Lazarus for the dead, He called him forth. It says that he who died came forth bound hand and foot, and his face was wrapped. Then Jesus said for those nearby to set him free.

> John 11:44
> And he who had died came out bound hand and foot with graveclothes, and his face was wrapped with a cloth. Jesus said to them, "Loose him, and let him go."

Sometimes it's like that when people get saved. They have new life given to them from Christ, but sometimes need help to no longer be in bondage. Their identity is changed at salvation, and it will fully be apparent as they start to walk out their freedom in Christ. Even though one's new identity may not be fully apparent (manifested in action), it doesn't mean they are the same old person. Too often Christians are hindered by the enemy by believing the lie that their identity still lies in their past, primarily based on their previous failures. If they have a time of failure, the enemy is quick to say, "See, you are the same old person." What they need to remember is that their identity is not based on what they do, but on what God has done. The Bible says they are born again - a new creation in Christ. So, the lies of the enemy need to be taken captive quickly and broken off. When the enemy lies and says something like, "You are no different; you aren't qualified; you aren't loved, etc.", the person needs to immediately not receive those thoughts (take captive), and then state the opposite out loud such as, "Jesus loves me so much

He died for me; there is no condemnation for those in Christ; I'm a new creation in Christ, etc." Sometimes a person will tend to believe a lie without realizing it. It might be influenced by their upbringing or childhood events. For example, if they were raised without a father, they may think their heavenly father doesn't really have much interest in them. If they were raised by a dominating mother, they may think the Holy Spirit, who is supposed to be our nurturer and comforter, is a task master. So, they may need help identifying the lie. Once they acknowledge it, they should say out loud that they break agreement with the lie, and then speak the truth. It's often good for them to ask the Holy Spirit what the truth is. Make sure it makes sense. The enemy may try to pretend to be the Holy Spirit if they aren't used to the Holy Spirit's voice.

In each case where someone feels oppressed, there are basically one to three steps to freedom. In the event that the enemy has no legal right to afflict a person, then the enemy can simply be commanded to leave in Jesus name. For cases where the demonic has a right, or at least believe they do, it will be a two or three step process to get rid of them.

For those situations where the enemy believes he has a right, we often call this a stronghold. I've heard the analogy of a mountain climber used. If a mountain climber is just climbing free handed, he could easily be knocked off the mountain. However, in the case where the climber looks for cracks to hammer in a pylon to attach to the mountain, he then will be difficult to knock off since he has something to hold on to. This is the case with the demonic. Thus, we use the phrase, "having an attachment." So, in this case the steps to freedom are to first break the attachment, and then second command the enemy to leave. I've seen cases where the first step is skipped, and by brute force the enemy is removed. The problem with that is the root has not been dealt with, and I find that in most cases the enemy is back the next day.

11

The attachments come in three ways. They can come by an action one does themselves. It can be an action someone else has done. Lastly, it can be generational. Each of these three can be broken down into subcategories such as sinful patterns, believing lies of the enemy, words spoken over us, unforgiveness, generational curses, dealing with the occult, and more. In every case it starts by understanding the reason for the stronghold which I will address in the rest of the book.

In general, the steps to freedom for each of the three avenues to the attachments listed above are as follows:

- If caused by self – repent, renounce, then cast off
- If caused by others – break off the power and effect, then cast off
- If generational – plead the blood of Jesus over your ancestral line, then cast off

Let me explain a few of these terms. Repentance is a term most people that grew up around the church understand. It's having a change in mind that changes direction. It makes way for grace. Usually, it begins with confession. This is a confession of wrong doing to God, and in return He forgives us. When we receive His forgiveness, our relationship is healed.

When we say we renounce something, we are telling the demonic that we no longer will have anything to do with that thing or activity we are renouncing. This severs their right to afflict due to an activity we were engaged in.

Casting off is just what it says. Removing the demon by commanding it to leave. When it comes to the casting off, or out, the demon, I'll command it to leave in Jesus name, and I'll usually just tell it to go wherever Jesus tells it to go. However, if it's very rebellious, difficult, and especially if it's been violent, I'll ask Jesus to have it sent to the abyss or straight to hell. It's not that I don't trust Jesus, but our opinions matter. You may ask why I don't send them all to the abyss. I just find it easier to tell them to go where Jesus tells them to go. I care more about the freedom of the person than the immediate future of the demonic. So, that's my primary focus. That is, until the demonic don't want to leave without a fight.

If you're wondering what may be a basis for sending them to the abyss, for that I have two reference points. The first being that sometimes I'll ask the person to ask Jesus where the demon was sent, and they will sometimes say it was sent to hell or the abyss. The second being that the demonic know that this is a possibility as we can see in the story of the demon-possessed man in the Gadarenes.

> Luke 8:30-31
> 30 Jesus asked him, saying, "What is your name?" And he said, "Legion," because many demons had entered him. 31 **And they begged Him that He would not command them to go out into the abyss.**

The stronghold can come from many other sources besides what we may have opened the door to. The specific type of stronghold can be revealed by a simple interview process. You can ask the one you are ministering to when it all started. Ask the Holy Spirit to bring things to their mind. Also, the one ministering the deliverance and those interceding should keep listening to the Holy Spirit for information and direction.

Matthew 12:29 talks about binding the strongman. The enemy can be bound with our authority. You could say that is like placing him under arrest (using the analogy of the police officer). This is important to do at the very beginning so they don't interfere in the process leading up to them being cast out or off. Make sure that the person being ministered to knows that you are talking to the enemy and not them. Then bind the enemy and command them to be silent

13

and not interfere. Again, this step is very important as they otherwise will interfere or lie to the person and may even pretend to be the Holy Spirit. This will be obvious by what they say they are hearing.

One of my very first deliverances was for a teenage boy who had tried to commit suicide. At first, the session was going very slowly because his responses to my questions were very slow. So, I asked him why it was taking so long to answer my questions. He said because every time I asked him a question, they (the demonic) would start talking to him. So, once I became aware of that, I commanded them to be silent and stop interfering in Jesus name. The session then went very quick as the Holy Spirit helped me discover the root of the issue. Once we dealt with the root cause, I commanded the demonic to go wherever Jesus told them to go.

I would also point out that I personally don't like to interview the demonic. There is some value to know the type of demon that is involved. For one thing, you will know what the activity was that opened the door to him. There is also something about commanding a specific type out that seems to be more effective. I know that is why some people do ask the demonic for their functional name, but as a general rule, I don't. They will often give themselves away by what they say that is not solicited. For example, a generational demon might burst out that he's been there forever.

Another part of the interview process is getting to know the person's testimony. It's important that they either are a Christian or are willing to become one, or things could get worse.

> Luke 11:24-26
> 24 "When an unclean spirit goes out of a man, he goes through dry places, seeking rest; and finding none, he says, 'I will return to my house from which I came.' 25 And when he comes, he finds it swept and put in order. 26 Then he goes

14

and takes with him seven other spirits more wicked than himself, and they enter and dwell there; and the last state of that man is worse than the first."

In this scripture we see the need to fill that which has been vacated. So, the very first thing we need to be sure of before anyone can be free of the demonic is that they are saved. So, in a sense you could say I never cast demons out of an unsaved person. I start with making sure the person is saved. If there is any doubt in my mind, I will walk them through what I would call a renewing of one's vows. Like with marriage there are times a couple will choose to renew their vows. This can be done for a good marriage, but it's especially important if there had been problems in their marriage. So, I use that analogy when walking a person through a renewing of making a covenant with Jesus for their salvation.

I've been fortunate to have had the opportunity to lead many to Christ as their Savior when they have come to me for freedom. I'll usually start our sessions by getting to know them, and part of that is understanding their spiritual background. If it's obvious to them and me that they have not ever received Christ as their Savior, I'll lead them into that great exchange. Deliverance can start right there. You can explain how if we confess we are sinful and in need of a savior, believe Jesus came to die to save us from our sins, and choose to repent from our sinfulness, He will exchange His righteousness for our sin. That is, He will remove our sin and give us a new spirit that is sinless.

TAKING THE ENEMY TO COURT – BREAKING GENERATIONAL CURSES AND COVENANTS

Some will talk about the courtroom of heaven and spiritually going there for declaring freedom. I too have found this to be effective for particular situations. Where I believe this to be most useful is when it comes to one's generational bloodline. In one's family, generations in the past may have made unholy dedications and unholy covenants. These covenants can affect future generations until they are broken.

You don't necessarily need to state you are entering the courtrooms of heaven, but in some cases I feel it appropriate and powerful. Sometimes I simply state that I'm pleading the blood of Christ for some situation. That statement implies legal action, like that of pleading something before a judge. So, I will say something along the lines of, "I plead the blood of Christ to create a wall of separation between myself and all previous generations, removing the right of the demonic to afflict me due to any of their sinful actions. I remove all unholy things and only allow righteous things to be passed through my bloodline in Jesus name." There are times I will do this one generation at a time back four generations, and then a general one after that if I feel led to do so. The reason I choose four

16

generations is because in the books of Numbers and Deuteronomy it says the children will suffer the sins up to the third and fourth generation. While this is in the old covenant, the demonic don't care. The demonic are very legalistic, and they will try to use God's word to find where they might be able to use it against us. So, I will proceed to remove any area that they think they have legal ground until they realize they have none. For example, when my wife and I were on a missions trip in Myanmar, a lady asked us to pray for her daughter. Her daughter had been having demonic visitations at night and was tormented. Having Buddhist heritage prior to her Christian parents, I pleaded the blood of Christ over her and removed the right of the demonic to afflict her because of previous generations' sin. I chose to do this one generation at a time. When I did the grandparents' generation, something powerful happened, and she fell against me. I held her up and quickly finished. She awoke and had a huge smile on her face. She told her mom that she felt great. We all knew that she had been set free.

There was another time when I was leading a lady through a similar prayer taking one generation at a time. Some of her family had been in the occult. When I got to the grandparents' generation, she stopped repeating me. I kept waiting, and she signaled she couldn't talk. The demonic were restricting her vocal chords. They knew it would remove any right that they had. I quickly commanded them to release her voice and not interfere in Jesus name. We then continued, and I cast them off of her.

One severely demonized teen that I ministered to had a mix of doors she had opened herself to as well as occult involvement in her family. In her case I dealt with the doors she personally opened first. I then entered the courtroom of heaven on her behalf for the occult involvement of her family. I needed to break unholy vows and covenants in her generational line, and I felt it best to do in the courtroom of heaven. It proved to be very effective, and then the demonic were easy to remove.

Here are some suggested prayers for generational curses and covenants.

In the name of Jesus, I plead the blood of Jesus to create a wall of separation between myself and all previous generations all the way back to Adam. I remove every right of the demonic to afflict me because of any previous generation's sin, but I call forth all righteous inheritance coming to me in Jesus name.

Lord, I enter your courtroom now, and I plead the blood of Christ to nullify and void any unholy covenant, contract, or agreement in my bloodline. I remove every right for the enemy to afflict me or my family due to all covenants, contracts, and agreements made by previous generations in Jesus name.

I now command any unholy spirit attached to my bloodline to leave and go wherever Jesus tells you to go in Jesus name.

TAKING THOUGHTS CAPTIVE AND BREAKING EMOTIONAL STRONGHOLDS

Inner healing is a term we give to healing your soul. We are made in God's image. Just as there are three parts of God: Father, Son (Jesus), and Holy Spirit, there are three parts of us: spirit, soul, and body. Our body gives us an awareness of the physical world around us. Our soul is made up of our mind and emotions. Our spirit is the part of us that allows us to have an awareness and connection with God. It is the part of us that is immediately made new when we accept Jesus as our savior.

> 2 Corinthians 5:17
> 17 Therefore, if anyone is in Christ, he is a new creation; old things have passed away; behold, all things have become new.

The moment we accept Christ, our spirits become brand new and connected with the Holy Spirit. The enemy can, however, afflict our bodies and souls to try and quench our spirit.
So, what we need to realize is that it's a spiritual battle.

2 Corinthians 10:3-5
3 For though we walk in the flesh, we do not war according to the flesh. 4 For the weapons of our warfare are not carnal but mighty in God for pulling down strongholds, 5 casting down arguments and every high thing that exalts itself against the knowledge of God, bringing every thought into captivity to the obedience of Christ,

Compare those verses to Ephesians 6:10-12.

Ephesians 6:10-12
10 Finally, my brethren, be strong in the Lord and in the power of His might. 11 Put on the whole armor of God, that you may be able to stand against the wiles of the devil. 12 For we do not wrestle against flesh and blood,

The first step to victory is to fight the right enemy. I know this sounds obvious, but you'd be surprised how many Christians are not doing that. Our battle is not against flesh. This includes ourselves. Our battle is against principalities, against powers, against the rulers of the darkness of this age, against spiritual hosts of wickedness in the heavenly places.

Since our war is not fleshly, we need our weapons to not be carnal. While pills may help with some symptoms, they won't solve a spiritual issue. First, let me say, if you are one of the many struggling with emotional issues requiring medication, I don't want you to feel condemned. In fact, I will never recommend anyone to get off of their medication without the approval of their doctor. I once helped a man get free of depression, and he asked if he should stop taking his medication. I told him to work that out with his doctor, and with the doctor's approval he was able to ween off of it.

I was reading an article several months ago on the pharmaceutical industry. To my shock, according to <u>Money</u> magazine nearly 20% of American adults have a diagnosable mental, emotional, or behavioral problem. I would say the enemy is being pretty effective in keeping people in bondage.

When they think of the demonic, most people probably tend to think of third world pagan countries. That makes sense. The demonic tends to be more blatant there. But I'll tell you, the demonic is very active in America. The problem is we tend to not notice it as demonic. Most of the time it comes in the form of negative emotions and irrational or tormenting thoughts. This is a spiritual issue, and this realization alone is very helpful.

For example, in my past I had seasons of depression. However, once I learned how to fight it, it ended. See, in the past I would ask God to help me to be free of my depression - to heal me of my depression. The problem with doing that is that I would own it. Something was wrong with me. I'm the problem. Meanwhile the enemy sits back and is really not affected much by my prayers, at least not long term. However, once I realized it's not me, but a spirit radiating his emotions onto me, I was able to walk in freedom because I could place the fight where it needed to be.

Your soul can be joyful, prosperous, and it can glorify God. It should be these things if you are saved because the Holy Spirit lives in you producing the fruit of the Spirit which are love, joy, peace, etc. However, our souls can also be sick, wounded, stressed, etc. As Christians, we have rivers of living water that flow out of our bellies.

> John 7:38
> He who believes in Me, as the Scripture has said, out of his heart will flow rivers of living water.

That just sounds refreshing to me. It also makes me think of the first part of Psalm 23:3.

> Psalm 23:3 New International Version (NIV)
> He refreshes my soul.
> He guides me along the right paths for his name's sake.

Sometimes our souls need to be refreshed, and the Holy Spirit brings refreshment to our souls. We see times in the Bible where angels also minister to our souls. We see this with Jesus in the garden.

> Luke 22:43
> Then an angel appeared to Him from heaven, strengthening Him.

Our souls can also be oppressed: attacked by the enemy. This is important to realize because it can affect your body and your spirit. Since your soul is in the center between your body and spirit, it is usually his primary target.

The Bible is clear that as Christians we are all capable of overcoming the enemy.
However, a lot of Christians have faith in the finished work of the cross to get them to heaven when they die, but are trying to do life on their own here on earth. So, I want to tell you, what you have probably already realized, it doesn't work.

Jesus did a lot more for you than just get you out of hell. He exchanges His righteousness for your sin. He suffered to exchange His healing for your sickness. He exchanges His glory for your shame. I could go on, but the point is He desires for you to live in victory and prosperity in this life, and He has made provision to do so.

Most parents want their kids to be successful in what they do. They want them to prosper. Likewise, our heavenly Father wants us to prosper in this life: in our health, in our job, in our ministry, in our relationships.

> 3 John 2
> Beloved, I pray that you may prosper in all things and be in health, just as your soul prospers.

> Or as the King James translation put it:
> Beloved, I wish above all things that you may prosper, and be in health, even as your soul prospers.

Look at it this way, God desires that you not have a messed up life. See, the problem is when you have an unhealthy soul, it can affect all areas of your life. It can affect your physical health, your emotions, your finances, your relationships, and more. You need to know that it's the desire of the heart of your Father in Heaven that you prosper (that is do well) in all things, and to do that you need to get rid of the junk in your soul.

Our souls can get full of all kinds of junk from what we watch, what we listen to, what activity we partake in, etc. We can also just let our emotions be vulnerable to the enemy which can bring fear, anxiety, depression, and other emotional disorders.

Now again, as a Christian we have the Holy Spirit in us who produces His fruit of love, joy, peace, patience, etc. These are what we as Christians should be walking in. The reason many of us don't experience the life God is intending for us is we don't know how to get rid of the junk in our soul and fight the enemy.

Have you ever been in a room where someone full of agitation walks in, and you can feel it radiating from him? It's the same way with the demonic. They are full of fear, anxiety, and depression, and they try to radiate that onto you. Sometimes we open doors to them by where we go, what we do, what we watch, or what we listen to.

Sometimes we haven't done anything wrong; just living in this world can be enough.

So again, if you are praying for God to fix your issue of depression or anxiety, you are missing the fact that it's not your problem. Instead you need to realize it's a spirit harassing you. Once you realize that, getting rid of it is easy.

I remember one time my wife and I were invited to come to a house hosting a small group to minster in healing. We saw God show up in a powerful way, and people got healed. After a few people got healing of some physical ailments, we asked one lady if there was anything she wanted prayer for. She replied that she didn't know if we could help her, but she was desperately wanting to be healed of depression. The problem was she didn't know that it was an oppressing spirit. She just thought it was a different form of physical healing that was needed even though it was a mental or emotional problem. Healing her was actually quite easy because we knew that it was a spirit of depression. Physically she was fine, but she was being harassed by a spirit. We simply commanded it to go in Jesus name, and it left. We then taught her how she could do the same by simply using the authority she had in her identity in Christ with the power of the name of Jesus.

I want to point out that often circumstances create situations in our lives that will make the attack of the enemy more likely to be effective. I'll give you an example from 2nd Timothy. This is the second epistle (that is book of the New Testament in the form of a letter) written from Paul to his spiritual son Timothy.

The timing of this is such that Paul is thrown in a dungeon of sorts for his ministry, facing death, and he is urging Timothy to be faithful regardless of the hardships the ministry might bring. This is in the realm of true persecution for one's faith. You can see how the surroundings may be intimidating to a young minister of the gospel.

> 2 Timothy 1:6
> Therefore, I remind you to stir up the gift of God which is in you through the laying on of my hands.

Paul reminds him of his purpose. Let me say that we all have a purpose.

Then Paul gives the contrast of what a Christian **might** feel or be moved by, to what a Christian **should** feel and be moved by.

> 2 Timothy 1:7
> For God has not given us a spirit of fear, but of power and of love and of a sound mind.

Here we see the mention of a spirit of fear. When fear or anxiety becomes the driving force in your life, when it becomes irrational, you are most likely being driven by a spirit of fear. So, as I already mentioned, the demonic can radiate this type of emotion onto you. A spirit of fear radiates fear that can get on you, which results in oppression. In this case, I feel the concern is that a spirit of fear is trying to quench Timothy's ministry.

Fear is also a doorway to other problems. One time a lady brought her mother to us for prayer because she had been diagnosed with pancreatic cancer. Before we prayed for the cancer, I opened in prayer and asked God to direct our time together. I immediately got a picture of a rawhide dog bone. Rawhide dog bone? I obviously thought that was a strange thing to see. However, I've learned that it's the thoughts and pictures that are the strangest in the present context that I've found the most valuable. So, I asked if they happened to have a dog that they give rawhide dog bones to as a treat sometimes. They said oh yes, and the dog loved them. They went on to say how they loved that dog very much. I noticed they referred to the dog in past tense. So, I asked what had happened to the dog. They said it died of pancreatitis. It suffered greatly, and the daughter said that her mother got fearful of ever suffering like that when she watched her dog suffer.

The lady's fear had opened a door to the very thing she feared. After a little more discussion it became apparent that she was also afraid of death. She wasn't confident of her eternal destination. So, we proceeded to share the gospel, and she received Jesus as her savior. We then broke off the fear that came on her from watching her dog suffer, and then prayed for her healing. We had a follow up report months later that she was doing fine.

Fear, anxiety, and other emotional afflictions are bad in themselves. If these are left unaddressed, they can open up the oppressed person to larger issues. Stress is a huge door to physical affliction. Again, the issue starts in the soul and later will often manifest in the body. Even doctors know the impact of stress on one's health. They would encourage lifestyle changes and stress management exercises. But, as Christians, we have much more to access for true healing.

So, what does Paul say to Timothy besides that God has not given him a spirt of fear? God has given you a Spirit of power. What kind of power? The kind with which Jesus did miracles. The kind that rose Jesus from the dead! The dunamis power I spoke of previously.

He's given you a Spirit of love. And as the Bible says, perfect love casts out all fear.

Lastly, the Spirit is one of a sound mind. When your mind is being tormented, it's listening to the wrong voice. The enemy will speak to you to the point where you start believing things that don't even make sense.

Back to Ephesians 6.

13 Therefore take up the whole armor of God, that you may be able to withstand in the evil day, and having done all, to stand.

14 Stand therefore, having girded your waist with truth, having put on the breastplate of righteousness, 15 and having shod your feet with the preparation of the gospel of peace; 16 above all, taking the shield of faith with which you will be able to quench all the fiery darts of the wicked one.

17 And take the helmet of salvation, and the sword of the Spirit, which is the word of God;

Verses 13-17 discuss the armor of God. I'm not going to go through that right now.

However, the sword is very important for this discussion. First, note that it's the Holy Spirit's sword. So, to use it properly, you should use it in conjunction with Him (the Holy Spirit). This is very apparent when you look at the Greek word and realize that it's *rehma* and not *logos*.

Rehma is the Greek word for the direct word from the Lord. Usually it's a truth that needs to be revealed. It will often contain logos (written word of God), but is a message particular to that situation. That being said, filling our heads with God's Word is of vital importance. We receive it from reading, meditating, memorizing, and hearing God's Word. James says to sing Psalms - sing praises. Have you ever had a song get stuck in your head? What we listen to all the time will start to influence our thoughts and behavior without us even being aware of it.

We need to realize that many strongholds are built on top of lies. This is why 2 Corinthians 10:5 says to take every thought captive. Many of those thoughts are lies placed there by the enemy. These can be lies you have come to believe about yourself, others (spouse, family, etc.), God, or a specific situation. The crazy thing is that the lie can be very irrational, but when placed in your mind in the right circumstance, you will consider it. Then it's like a snow ball; the more you let it roll around in your mind the larger it becomes. That's why you need to take those thoughts captive before they grow into strongholds. Strongholds of thought lead to strongholds of behavior. Even in the natural, disobedience starts with not listening or listening to the wrong source.

Some examples of irrational thoughts or emotions are as follows:
- Irrational fear
- Constant anxiety
- Suicidal thoughts
- Constant anger
- Built up hatred toward self or others
- Acts of self-harm (cutting, suicide)

The above list is more extreme manifestations of irrational thoughts, but they can also present in ways such as:
- Not feeling loved
- Thinking no one likes you
- Having a low self-image
- Feeling like you're always left out or over-looked

The Holy Spirit, however, gives you a sound mind. He helps you see things correctly. So, ask God what lie you are believing. It may be about yourself, about others, about Him, or about a situation. Take time to listen, but it shouldn't take long for the Holy Spirit to reveal one if it's there. Then ask Him for the truth. Then state the truth about that situation out loud. This is using the Sword of the Spirit. It diffuses the power of those lies. Many times the truth will be accompanied by a verse or a piece of scripture, but the important thing to know is that God is speaking directly to that situation.

Here are some suggested prayers to say out loud for freedom from emotional affliction and the breaking belief of lies.

I command depression, anxiety, fear, and hatred off of me in Jesus name.

I choose to break agreement with the lie that _____.

Some examples of lies to fill in that blank would be God doesn't love me, nobody cares about me, I'm a mistake, I'm not worthy of forgiveness, etc.

So now you know how to get rid of the bad emotions (fear, anxiety, depression, etc.), but how about receiving the good (love, joy, peace, etc.)? What if you could take a pill that produced the feeling of peace or joy, or wouldn't it be crazy if it made you feel loved? That pill would be a best seller. But you don't need to take a pill. Love, joy, and peace are fruit of the Holy Spirit. In fact, Romans 15 refers to God as the God of comfort (vs 5), the God of hope (vs 13), and the God of peace (vs 33).

When you say "the god of something", it typically is in charge of producing that item. For example, in Greek mythology, a god of rain produces rain. Of course that is all fake, nothing but false gods. But the one true God is also referred to as the God of comfort, hope, and peace because that is what He is known for producing. For the Christian, **that** God lives inside of you! So, how do you access what is being produced by the Holy Spirit? Ask for it.

Here is a simple prayer example for being filled with God's peace:

Holy Spirit I ask that you fill me with more of your fruit of peace in Jesus name.

You could do the same for joy or another fruit of the Spirt as well.

THE POWER OF WORDS

I was at a conference where the speaker said that he felt we should pray for those with hearing problems. A lady in the row behind me got up, and those of us gathered around her, laid hands on her, and prayed. She looked to be in her 60's, so it didn't surprise me that she had hearing problems. When we finished praying, everyone started going back to their seats, but I really felt the presence of God so I asked her if she noticed any difference. She took out her hearing aids and said no; there was no difference. So, I asked if I could pray again. I laid hands on her ears and prayed for healing. I felt the presence of God so strong my faith was really high. I asked again, but she said no change. Normally, I would just stop and bless her at this point, but the presence of God was so strong I really expected some change. So, I asked her to tell me about when her hearing problems began. She said that ever since she was a little girl she had hearing problems. She shared some medical background and trouble as a child with ears including blistering. Then she caught my attention with the next statement. She said that her mother said that she would have hearing problems the rest of her life. I immediately responded with asking if I could pray again. I said, "In Jesus name I break off the words spoken over you by your mother, and I command the spirit of deafness to go." She fell back into her seat which I didn't expect. Then she had this perplexed look on her face which turned to joy, and she said, "The roaring is gone." I didn't know what she was talking about because she never mentioned a roaring before this. The reason she needed the hearing aids was to amplify the sound over the roar she had heard in her ears.

That night it hit me how, unfortunately, we are sometimes careless with our words as well. Our words can often do tremendous damage. We need to be careful with our tongues. We may not even realize the damage we are doing.

I had a teen come to me one time for prayer for his foot. Again, I had a situation where I felt the power of God present for healing, but nothing was happening. So, I quietly asked the Holy Spirit for revelation if something was blocking the healing. I then asked the young man when this all started. He mentioned it was during football. As we continued, it became apparent that this was a result of a soul wound. The coach was very hard on him, and it had a huge impact on him. When we dealt with the soul wound of the words spoken over him, healing started to take place for the foot.

I have been involved in jail ministry for many years. As you would expect, many of the inmates were told most all of their lives that they will be nothing but trouble. Sometimes words can come in the form of a label placed on a person such as fatty or stupid, etc. Sadly, these labels set a path for one's future when they are received. The labels can even be given by professionals such as doctors. Once a person is diagnosed with a disorder, they often resolve to accepting that is just who they are. Examples of this can be bipolar, hyperactive, or schizophrenic. While in some cases there may be a chemical disorder or something that needs to be physically corrected, there is usually a spiritual issue at the root. This can be generational or caused by a number of factors. Once the spiritual aspect is dealt with, there may be a need for prayer for the physical healing aspect as well.

One time when doing jail ministry, I was with one other guy visiting a cell pod. This particular night we had one inmate come to meet with us. When he realized he was going to be the only one, he said that he would be more open with us. He told us how he was diagnosed by doctors as being schizophrenic. No one had ever been able to help him, and he had even tried to kill himself. I told him that it was going to be the best day of his life. That was all about to change, and I led him through a deliverance session. The root of the problem was that he opened the door to the demonic 20 years ago while doing hallucinatory drugs. Since then he had all kinds of symptoms that were actually demonic manifestations. The doctors just throw labels on it because they aren't trained to heal spiritual issues. Unfortunately, he wasn't able to get help at the churches he visited either. As I led him through repentance and renouncing of the drug participation, he could already feel the demonic flying off of him. I then commanded the spirit of schizophrenia and anything still lingering to go. His joy was great as he finally felt free of all of the demonic oppression for the first time in 20 years.

Words that are received from authority figures have a strong impact. However, words that we speak over ourselves are just as dangerous. One minute you could be asking God to intervene on your behalf, but then a minute later you're cursing your situation. Many times we don't realize we are actually removing all power from our prayers in the process. Let's take finances for an example. Some may be praying for God to provide for them and help them in their time of need. Then later they will tell their friends on the phone how they're always poor. They would say how their whole family has always been poor. How their parents were poor, their grandparents were poor, and so on. Unknowingly, they are cursing the very situation they prayed about earlier.

Too often we curse our prayers. Pray what we want, but then later say how it will never happen. A person may say things like, "My husband or wife will never change." Another may actually be speaking to their body, cursing the parts that don't work right, don't look right, give them pain, etc.

What is in your heart will come out of your mouth. However, if you want to commit something to heart, you repeat something with your mouth. When you memorize something, it's easier to do that if you are processing it out loud, and when you're memorizing, you're saying you know it by heart, correct? This is why it's important to fill yourself with the Word of God, so you can have the proper perspective.

We may speak negatively over ourselves in what may seem like we are joking around. Sometimes we speak in frustration about a part of our body or over a situation we are in. The situation may be negative, but if we speak out loud about it, we can reinforce it with our words. That negative self-talk can be destructive. The words can reflect what is going on inside a person as well. A funny movie scene that portrays this is seen in the Christopher Robin movie. Winnie the Pooh wants to play the "say what you see" game. He says things like balloon, tree, and bird. Piglet says, "fear, anxiety." When it's Eeyore's turn, he says, "depression, disappointment." If a person is always talking negatively about things, chances are they have a lot of negative self-talk, belief, and attitude toward themselves and/or others.

> Matthew 15:11
> Not what goes into the mouth defiles a man, but what comes out of the mouth, this defiles a man.

Jesus explains this in verses 17-18

Matthew15:17-18
What goes into the mouth goes into the stomach and is eliminated.
But those things that proceed out of the mouth come from the heart, and they defile a man.

So, what you really need is to get your heart right and your mind renewed.

From the very beginning Satan attacked what God said to man because he knows that thoughts lead to actions. So, the power of words could also be looked at as the power of our thought life or beliefs. But when those thoughts come out of your mouth, there is more power added to them.

John 7:38
Whoever believes in me, as the scripture has said, "Out of his heart will flow rivers of living water."

If it's flowing from your heart, it should flow from your mouth.

There can be times where we even unintentionally speak a vow over ourselves. One time when praying for a lady whose eyesight was degrading, I could sense a resistance. When I asked when it all started, a memory came back to her. She had a family member who was abusive to her and others in her family. This created bitterness in her, which alone can create health issues, but she remembered one time thinking about him in the car and saying out loud, "I'd rather go blind than forgive him!" From that point on her eyesight started to deteriorate. To deal with this, she needed to repent from speaking those words over herself. She also needed to forgive her relative for all he did. This is an act of the will because the emotions will resist. This by no means justifies his action, makes it okay, or means relationship or trust needs to be restored. It means none of that. It's simply releasing the bitterness and debt she feels is owed to her. Then hand the situation over to God for His righteous judgment. That's His role, not ours. I then broke the power of those words she spoke over herself in Jesus name. This made a way for healing to start, and we immediately started seeing progress.

Even the world recognizes the power of our tongues. Years ago I was at an extended family gathering, and we were playing Trivial Pursuit, a game that was popular at the time. We were divided into two teams. When it was our team's turn, we got the question, "what is the most powerful muscle?" We all turned to my cousin who was an orthopedic surgeon for the answer, but the answer wasn't looking just at mere physical strength. It was the tongue.

Proverbs 18:21 says we hold the power of life and death in our tongues. It doesn't get any stronger than that.

To visualize this, I was part of an online class where they taught on the power of words, and we did an experiment with two jars of cooked rice. For about a week we spoke nicely to one of the jars every day, and the other we spoke harshly to every day. The jar that we spoke nicely to stayed looking healthy, while the jar of rice we spoke harshly to started turning black.

Jesus cursed the fig tree, and it withered. We tend to think of curses in the negative sense, and for the most part that is true. However, there have been times I've cursed cancer or a disease, and I believe it assisted prayers for healing. Curses can be intentional or unintentional. There are times curses can be put on a person. Sometimes it can simply be words spoken against a person in hatred with intent to do harm. I know it seems hard to believe, but that was the root cause of a woman's cancer for whom I was praying for once. Breaking off the words spoken over her made way for physical healing.

There was a time I even came across a case of a witch doctor's curse when praying for a man's eye. He had an eye that had gone completely blind. A doctor had diagnosed the problem as a result of a blood clot behind the eye. As I prayed, the man said he felt life coming back to his eye, and he began to see shadows. Unfortunately, that was as far we got that night. I ran into him a year later and asked about his eye. It was the same. No better. No worse. I invited him to come over for lunch the next Sunday, and I planned to pick him up after church. The night before our lunch plans, I woke up in the night, and I started praying for wisdom on how to pray for this man. I immediately saw the picture of a witch doctor's face in my mind's eye. So, when he was over, I told him what I saw and asked if this made any sense to him. He said he heard of a witch doctor in Africa, which is where he was from, placing curses on people. So, I broke off the power of that curse in Jesus name. He immediately got super excited because he felt something come off of his chest that had been plaguing him for years. He started praising God and said he wanted to stand on my roof top praising God. I then prayed for his eye, and he started seeing color. It didn't reach full healing, but it did improve some more. He didn't even seem to care about his eye anymore relative to being set free from what was on his chest.

Here is an example of how to break off the power of words or curses:

I break off any spell, curse, incantation, or words spoken against me in Jesus name. I declare that they will all fall powerless to the ground in Jesus name.

I break off the words that _____ spoke over me in Jesus name.

I choose not to receive the words _____ spoke over me.

BREAKING SINFUL PATTERNS AND ADDICTIVE STRONGHOLDS

I have done jail ministry over many years now, and as you can imagine, drug and alcohol addiction are very common problems among the inmates. I could say that addiction to pornography is also a common issue, but that's a huge issue outside of jail as well, including within the church. So, I've always found the subject of dealing with addictions especially interesting since I strongly desired a good solution to offer those deep in bondage.

Historically, the church has taught solutions that help manage the symptoms of a deeper issue. There is actually great wisdom in some of these teachings, such as changing your environment and even your friends, in some cases. For example, for an alcoholic to continue to hang out at bars with friends that entice him to drink would be foolish. However, one may find themselves becoming a closet alcoholic trying to keep a certain appearance and avoid judgement from others. This example, of course, could be for any addictive behavior. Accountability often will only make addicts into liars as well so they can avoid the shame often used to manipulate them into behaving a certain way. In fact, in my parents' generation, the phrase "shame on you" was commonly used. Without knowing it, they were opening the person's soul up to be oppressed by a spirit of shame.

To say this is a spiritual issue may seem obvious, but it's not usually addressed that way. We would get the person saved, and then we expected them to discipline the flesh to overcome their sin and strongholds. I first want to say that I by no means want to downplay the power of one's salvation. In fact, I've seen times when a person gets saved and are immediately delivered from all addictions. However, that's not always the case, and the power of the cross needs to be applied properly to set them free. What Jesus did on the cross is enough, period. All the benefits of His death are not always received automatically, but they're all presently available.

There seems to be a thought in the church that if a person is truly a Christian he shouldn't struggle with sin. There is Biblical truth to back that up. Christians are overcomers. Christians don't regularly practice sin. Christians have been set free from the bondage of sin. Christians have been transformed to a whole new creation. I could go on. However, the problem comes from a lack of understanding. Our spirit man has been completely sanctified and transformed, but our soul is in the process of being sanctified. Like muscle memory we need our souls to be retrained. But even a bigger difference is that the enemy has no access to the spirit of a Christian. The spirit of a Christian is intertwined with the Holy Spirit. A Christian's soul, on the other hand, can be influenced by the enemy to the point of a stronghold until we deal with it.

So, the longer a person has been a Christian, the harder it will be for them to be open about their struggles. In order to actually help someone, they need to feel they can be totally honest without ever feeling judgement or shame. They need to know that's not really who they are. I'm not saying they don't own up to their actions, but it's not the core of their being. Their spirit wants to do what is right.

Peter is a perfect example of this. He was one of the most zealous of Jesus' disciples. Satan saw him as a threat which is why Jesus told Peter (Simon) that Satan has asked that Peter be sifted as wheat.

> Luke 22:31-32
> 31 And the Lord said, "Simon, Simon! Indeed, Satan has asked for you, that he may sift you as wheat. 32 But I have prayed for you, that your faith should not fail; and when you have returned to Me, strengthen your brethren."

You may think that Satan wanted to kill Peter, and he probably did want to kill him. However, Jesus predicts Peter's failure and that he will need to be restored. He then tells Peter, once you are restored (have returned to me), strengthen your brethren (verse 32). Why does He say this? He says this because He knows Peter is still to be a leader. His failure doesn't define who he is to be.

Jesus knows the power of shame, and it temporarily takes Peter out. Jesus in His divine wisdom recreates the scene to bring healing to that memory. He has Peter join him at a charcoal fire, reminiscent of the one he stood by when he denied the Lord. He then walks him through a healing process. He asks Peter three times if he loves Him. One time for each denial. I used to read that passage and thought it had to be miserable for Peter to keep being asked that, but Jesus must have known the healing power of asking him three times. Each time Peter answered that he did love Jesus, even if it wasn't as strong a term for love as Jesus asked. After each response of Peter, Jesus gave a commission of a Shepherd. Feed my lambs, tend my sheep, and feed my sheep. He affirmed to Peter that his purpose and calling hadn't changed.

All along, He keeps pulling Peter back to his calling. In Mark 16:7 Jesus tells Mary Magdalene to go tell the disciples and Peter. He made a point of calling out Peter's name. The scriptures also point out that Jesus visited Peter (Simon), implying a visit to him alone.

Luke 24:33-34

33 So they rose up that very hour and returned to Jerusalem, and found the eleven and those who were with them gathered together, 34 saying, "The Lord is risen indeed, **and has appeared to Simon!**"

So, Jesus makes sure Peter isn't taken out because of His failure. He restores Peter. He takes away the guilt and shame Peter is carrying that made him feel unworthy of ministry, much less leadership. Most importantly, I think Jesus showed Peter that his failure didn't define or change who he was in His eyes.

I'm not by any means saying it's okay to sin, or it won't affect your ministry. In fact, for those living in sin or in some kind of stronghold, they should take a break from ministry and get healthy.

So how do we help those who keep failing - those who are caught in strongholds and addictions? Well, as I already mentioned, we start by making sure they have received Jesus as their Savior, but next they need to ask Him to be Lord of their life. There are other exchanges we can make with Jesus after the great exchange that brings salvation. The main thing is to surrender things that the Lord is calling us to give up in our life. Often we need the power of God in order to give them up.

Let's take drug addiction as an example. To give up drug addiction, one should start with confession of turning to a substance rather than God for whatever they are trying to accomplish with the drug as a much inferior substitute. I remember one time when doing jail ministry asking the Holy Spirit to come on some inmates. One guy said that if he could feel like that all the time why would he ever want to take drugs. God brings genuine joy. After the confession of the choices, the person needs to ask for forgiveness, and then say they receive it. Have them say they receive the forgiveness out loud because this is very healing. It may be difficult for them to do because the enemy is accusing them and is bringing condemnation and guilt to their minds. They need to know and be reassured of how God sees them. He sees them as holy and washed clean. Next, they should confess any rebellious action and attitude they had and again receive God's forgiveness for that. Then we cleanse the soul by having them release all soul ties to whatever the addiction was. They should do that out loud. Lastly, they command the spirit of rebellion and any other pertinent spirits to leave them and never return. Examples of this may be addictive spirits, spirit of lust, or spirit of perversion. If the spirit tries to interfere, command it to stop, and if need be command it to leave for them.

Here is an example of steps for freedom from drug addiction, the door that it's opened, and the oppression as a result. This is to be done after any root issue has been addressed that may have led to the addiction such as trauma, lies believed about self, etc. (see other sections to address those doors).

Pray the following out loud:
- *Lord I confess my involvement with drugs, and I renounce doing drugs in Jesus name.*
- *I confess my rebellion in doing the drugs, and I renounce my rebellious attitude in Jesus name.*
- *I command any spirit of rebellion to leave me now and go wherever Jesus tells you to go in Jesus name.*
- *I command any spirit of addiction to leave me now and go wherever Jesus tells you to go in Jesus name.*
- *I command any spirits that I invited in through my involvement with drugs to leave me now and go wherever Jesus tells you to go in Jesus name.*

After steps for addictions are important. Provide those who were addicted with some declarations and verses to memorize. Have them place post it notes on their mirror or someplace else to remind them of who they are in Christ, etc.

Make sure whenever they fail, you choose to celebrate how long they successfully went since their last time. Pray with them, and break off any shame and guilt. Encourage them in the progress they are making. Ask the Holy Spirit to fill them up with peace. Break off any depression or other emotions the enemy is trying to bring. Again, you do this by commanding shame, guilt, and depression off of them in Jesus name.

BITTERNESS AND UNFORGIVENESS

Forgiveness is a huge factor when it comes to the demonic. If we harbor any bitterness toward someone and refuse to forgive them, we are vulnerable to all kinds of demonic torment. Jesus illustrates this in a parable about an unforgiving servant.

Matthew 18:21-35
21 Then Peter came to Him and said, "Lord, how often shall my brother sin against me, and I forgive him? Up to seven times?"
22 Jesus said to him, "I do not say to you, up to seven times, but up to seventy times seven. 23 Therefore the kingdom of heaven is like a certain king who wanted to settle accounts with his servants. 24 And when he had begun to settle accounts, one was brought to him who owed him ten thousand talents. 25 But as he was not able to pay, his master commanded that he be sold, with his wife and children and all that he had, and that payment be made. 26 The servant therefore fell down before him, saying, 'Master, have patience with me, and I will pay you all.' 27 Then the master

of that servant was moved with compassion, released him, and forgave him the debt.

28 But that servant went out and found one of his fellow servants who owed him a hundred denarii; and he laid hands on him and took him by the throat, saying, 'Pay me what you owe!' 29 So his fellow servant fell down at his feet and begged him, saying, 'Have patience with me, and I will pay you all.' 30 And he would not, but went and threw him into prison till he should pay the debt. 31 So when his fellow servants saw what had been done, they were very grieved, and came and told their master all that had been done. 32 Then his master, after he had called him, said to him, 'You wicked servant! I forgave you all that debt because you begged me. 33 Should you not also have had compassion on your fellow servant, just as I had pity on you?' 34 And his master was angry, and delivered him to the torturers until he should pay all that was due to him.

35 "So My Heavenly Father also will do to you if each of you, from his heart, does not forgive his brother his trespasses."

In this parable the King represents God the Father, and the debt is an analogy for our sin. Salvation is the largest act of forgiveness possible. So, like the unmerciful servant who had been forgiven much by the king, what right do we have to be unforgiving toward others?

In the parable it says the unforgiving servant was subject to the torturers. When we receive salvation, we are forgiven a huge debt. If we then refuse to forgive others after being forgiven so much by the Lord, we are susceptible to affliction by the enemy.

The enemy looks at this as legal access to torment those who refuse to have forgiving hearts toward others. This torment can manifest in a variety of ways, but often it's in the form of a physical infirmity.

As an example, I was leading a freedom session for a lady once, and as we often would do, we started by opening in prayer. When we did so, I immediately got a word of knowledge for back pain. I asked the lady if she had any back issues. She said, "Oh yes", and she lifted the bottom of her shirt to expose a back brace. So, I asked her if she had anyone she feels she needs to forgive, which would be a logical part of a freedom session anyway. Without hesitation she said that she did. So, we walked her through forgiving all of those that the Holy Spirit brought to mind to forgive. We then continued with the rest of the session, and I forgot all about her back. Then when she went to leave, she bent over to put on her shoes. Then with a smile she said, "It's been a long time since I've been able to bend over like this."

On a different occasion, I was praying for a lady's chronic pain in her forearms. At first one arm got a little better, but when praying for the other arm, it got much worse. In fact, she screamed and said, "Let me go." The fact was I was hardly touching her, but she needed deliverance. It turned out that she had unforgiveness toward her brother who would hold her down and torment her. This ended up manifesting as pain in her forearms.

When we harbor bitterness and unforgiveness, it can lead to other sinful mindsets and actions as well. For example, our pride may make us resentful for not being recognized or treated with proper respect. This can be seen in the actions of Simon the sorcerer.

> Acts 8:9-25
> 9 But there was a certain man called Simon, who previously practiced sorcery in the city and astonished the people of Samaria, claiming that he was someone great, 10 to whom they all gave heed, from the least to the greatest, saying, "This man is the great power of God." 11 And they heeded him because he had astonished them with his sorceries for a long time. 12 But when they believed Philip as he preached the things concerning the kingdom of God and the name of

Jesus Christ, both men and women were baptized. 13 Then Simon himself also believed; and when he was baptized he continued with Philip, and was amazed, seeing the miracles and signs which were done.

14 Now when the apostles who were at Jerusalem heard that Samaria had received the word of God, they sent Peter and John to them, 15 who, when they had come down, prayed for them that they might receive the Holy Spirit. 16 For as yet He had fallen upon none of them. They had only been baptized in the name of the Lord Jesus. 17 Then they laid hands on them, and they received the Holy Spirit.
18 And when Simon saw that through the laying on of the apostles' hands the Holy Spirit was given, he offered them money, 19 saying, "Give me this power also, that anyone on whom I lay hands may receive the Holy Spirit."
20 But Peter said to him, "Your money perish with you, because you thought that the gift of God could be purchased with money! 21 You have neither part nor portion in this matter, for your heart is not right in the sight of God. 22 Repent therefore of this your wickedness, and pray God if perhaps the thought of your heart may be forgiven you. 23 For I see that **you are poisoned by bitterness and bound by iniquity.**"
24 Then Simon answered and said, "Pray to the Lord for me, that none of the things which you have spoken may come upon me."
25 So when they had testified and preached the word of the Lord, they returned to Jerusalem, preaching the gospel in many villages of the Samaritans.

After Simon got saved, he saw the power of the Holy Spirit come on others through the laying on of the apostles' hands, and he asked if he could buy that gift. Peter responded with insight that Simon had been "poisoned by bitterness and bound by iniquity." He was still

46

bound after his salvation. As a result, his "heart was not right in the sight of God." So, most likely Simon's motivation for the gift was to exalt himself. However, the root of this was bitterness.

Sometimes bitterness can take time to be rid of. Therefore, like any unforgiveness, it is an act of the will to choose to do it. The emotions will need to follow the decision, not drive it.

To clarify any misunderstanding, forgiveness is a releasing of a debt. It's choosing to have the attitude that they don't owe me anything. It's not saying that the offense was okay. It's not deciding to reestablish trust (that needs to be earned). It's not even saying that one is to pursue relationship again with the person that hurt them. It's simply choosing to let go of the offense.

To do this, say out loud (so the enemy can hear it), *I choose as an act of my will to forgive _____ for _____. I release them to you Lord Jesus for your righteous judgement and blessing.*

Soul Ties

Soul ties are persons, places, or things that have a connection to a person's soul to the point of influence. In the case of substance addiction, you could say they have a soul tie to that substance. That was covered when we discussed addictive strongholds. I want to focus more in this chapter about soul ties to other people.

Soul ties can be good or bad. Usually they are developed in the case of sexual relations. This is part of God's design since he intended for a monogamous sexual relationship between a man and a woman in the context of marriage, and the two are to become one. Unlike with animals, sex for humans is face to face. There is a soul connection with that physical connection, and during that time things attached to the souls are shared in the spiritual realm. This was meant to be a good thing. Unfortunately, it can have very negative effects when there is an unhealthy soul shared to another person's soul.

I remember a lady who came to us one time for freedom from chronic depression. I felt it came in through a soul tie. When I asked her about it, she realized that it all started back when she had sexual relations with a guy who himself was tormented in mind and full of depression. So, we broke the soul tie, commanded the depression off of her, and she was set free.

There are many other types of soul ties that aren't formed in that physical manner. For example, there can be soul ties with friends that have a strong emotional connection as well as soul ties with family members. I believe this is why there is such grieving when a loved one dies. It strongly affects the soul and even manifests in the body. I've seen this often come in the form of hair turning gray – or even falling out - when a parent or other loved one dies.

An example of a healthy soul tie between two friends would be Jonathan and David. It says in 1 Samuel 18:1 that the soul of Jonathan was knit to the soul of David, and Jonathan loved him as his own soul.

When ministering to some teens, I've seen soul ties have an effect, even when there was no physical relationship. One time we were asked to minister to a young teenage girl who had shut down emotionally, was in deep depression, and even had suicidal thoughts. She was so afflicted by depression she wouldn't talk. She would only nod or shake her head. Thankfully, the Holy Spirit helped us figure out that this came from a soul tie with a friend suffering similar emotions and sexual confusion. She was actually trying to help her friend get out of her depression, but instead it resulted in her getting influenced by the same spirits. Once we broke the soul ties with the friend, there was an immediate change. We were able to discuss things with her. This made the rest of the session go quickly, and as we commanded things to go, she was set completely free.

We have had a few cases where teens were afflicted with both sexual confusion and depression. One case that comes to mind involved a teen whose parents contacted us after he tried to commit suicide. It's interesting to me how in some cases one spirit opens the door to the next. Besides attempted suicide and sexual confusion, he struggled with pain in his head when his dad would try to pray with him or read the Bible within earshot. His situation also stemmed from a soul tie to a friend. Once the soul tie was broken, the spirits started afflicting pain in his head. I commanded them to leave, and they did. I then asked his dad to come read scripture to him, and it was a peaceful and loving time.

So, how does one break unhealthy soul ties? Here is an example prayer for a generic soul cleansing of unhealthy soul ties. *"In the name of Jesus, I break all unhealthy soul ties to any people, places, and addictions, and anything of the enemy. I renounce any association with any of those people or things having evil influence in my life. I am free, and I am whole in Jesus name!"* Then ask the Holy Spirit to fill you up.

An example of more specific and effective way to pray for soul ties to people would be as follows: *In the name of Jesus I break all soul ties with _____ (insert the person's name, or category of people if there have been many in the past). I send back any part of them I have taken, and I receive back any given or taken part of me, washed through the blood of Christ so that I may be made whole and complete in Jesus name.*

DEALING WITH PREVIOUS OCCULT ACTIVITY

It's sad how many people have dabbled in the occult. Typically, it is because they believed one of four lies.

The first lie is that it's all just innocent fun. They don't really understand that they are dealing with entities that are really evil and want them harmed, in bondage, tormented, and even dead. It's easy to find Ouija boards in many game stores. One day I was curious how they market such a thing. So, I picked it up to look at the back cover. I immediately felt the demonic getting all over me. I quickly set it down and commanded them all to get off me in Jesus' name. After they all went flying off, I got my wife and left. I don't normally curse people or places, nor do I condone that activity. Our job is to breakdown strongholds over people and places. This is one time that I did; I declared the store to go out of business in Jesus name.

Unfortunately, the fact that we have a good number of psychics in business shows how many people open themselves up through divination of some sort. I have met numerous people who have dabbled with Ouija boards or tarot cards. There were two different occasions where I heard about a group playing with the Ouija board

51

at a party, and when it was a particular person's turn to ask it a question, they asked who was controlling the board. In both cases the answer was the same. The board spelled out Satan. You may wonder why the demonic would be so willing to just state the truth in this case, but they know that many really don't have a proper view of the dangers of dealing with Satan.

Many are really just very ignorant of the source of power of psychics, fortunetellers, and their tools. I remember one young lady with 21 diagnosed issues who asked us for prayer. After praying for her healing to absolutely no avail, I asked the Holy Spirit to bring to mind anything we should know. She said immediately what came to mind when I prayed was that when she was a girl she wanted to know her future so she started playing with Tarot cards. Things started going downhill physically for her ever since.

The second lie that is often believed is that a certain practice is natural. Take Reiki, Therapeutic Touch, or energy healing for example. They think that it's just natural channeling of energy for healing, but if you look into it you will find that Reiki has its roots in the occult. Yoga poses that mimic the worship to Hindu gods, hypnosis, and transcendental meditation are other areas that may seem natural, but can open oneself up to demonic influence.

The third lie many will believe is that an ability is a God given gift. I know one lady that grew up in a home that did séances. She was given the ability to supernaturally draw beautiful pictures when the demonic took control of her hand. She was told that it was a gift from God. She later got into mind control and other things. Then one day the demonic turned on her. They told her to kill herself. In fact, they kept yelling it over and over. Then suddenly they stopped and were completely quiet. She asked them what happened, and they said that Jesus said they went too far. This was the first time she heard of Jesus. To make a long story short, this led to her becoming a Christian.

The fourth lie of the enemy is that it will allow them to be powerful and that Christians aren't. This comes in many different forms. Some may even have been raised in a church that doesn't think healing and the gifts of the Spirit are for today, and they will believe the lie that Christians are powerless. When they are introduced to the power of the enemy, they are drawn to the counterfeit because they haven't experienced the real.

As I've mentioned in the chapter on dealing with generational curses, the occult in the family bloodline is a big issue as well. However, it's not just that it comes through the family bloodline, but often the practices get passed on to the next generations as well.

Now, of course, the level to which individuals have opened themselves up to the occult or Satanism can vary significantly.

As with any sin, there needs to be confession, repentance, and renouncing of the involvement. Most Christians are familiar with confession and repentance. That gets you right with God. But before you can cast off the demonic, there needs to be renouncement that is done out loud. This removes their legal rights for them to stay. It's to be done out loud so they can hear it. With the occult there may also be a need for breaking any unholy covenants or contracts through the blood of Christ. This should also be done out loud. Then you command them to go wherever Jesus sends them in Jesus name.

Here is an example of steps for involvement with a Ouija board and tarot cards.

Pray the following out loud:
- *Lord I confess my involvement with using a Ouija board and tarot cards, and I renounce all of that activity and any other activity with the occult of any kind in Jesus name.*

- *I command any spirits that I invited in through my involvement with those items leave me now and go wherever Jesus tells you to go in Jesus name.*

Overcoming Effects of Past Trauma

Trauma can have a huge impact on a person's soul as well as their body. It should come as no surprise that spiritual trauma can impact a person, but I've been shocked at the spiritual impact physical trauma can have on a person's soul.

Spiritual or emotional trauma can come in many different forms. There have been times when a sense of abandonment that a person has as a child can create trauma leading to irrational fears and anxieties as an adult. The enemy is usually quick to create lies and form belief patterns in a person's life from this type of situation. For example, a child can be in the hospital which can be traumatic to start with, and if no one is there on a regular basis, the child can grow up with a fear of abandonment. In this case there is an important need to walk the person through breaking agreement with the lie that they can't trust God to not abandon them. Sometimes it is important to focus on a specific person of the trinity. The lie that other people close to them will abandon them needs to be broken as well.

When breaking agreement with a lie, it's best to have the person state out loud that they break agreement with the lie that they are choosing to no longer believe. For example, if they are irrationally believing that their spouse is going to leave them (have no basis for thinking that), then they should say out loud, "I choose to break agreement with the lie that my spouse is going to leave me." Then just keep breaking other lies they are believing, such as their spouse doesn't care about them, etc. Then command all the lies that they were believing to be powerless in Jesus name. This could apply to a child having anxiety that their parents are going to leave them as well. The reason this is important to do out loud is that there is power in hearing truth out loud and the demonic can hear it as well. The demonic can place thoughts into your mind or whisper in your ear, but they can't read your mind. They should then command all fear related to those lies to leave in Jesus name.

More intense spiritual trauma could come in the form of abuse as a child. This could be emotional, physical, sexual, or even Satanic. Satanic abuse could come in the form of night terrors, demonic visitations, or even Satanic ritual abuse. Typically, if a child experiences sexual abuse, this could open all kinds of demonic activity in their life. There will be a need to break off the trauma, forgive the person involved, and possibly more depending on the specific situation. If it's a relative, generational curses will also need to be broken. If it stems from Satanism or Masons in the family line, then generational curses need to be broken as well as breaking unholy covenants and dedications.

Some of the more severe abuses can create multiple personalities as a protective response of the mind. These personalities are sometimes referred to as parts. These parts are not demons, and one should not attempt to kick them out. While ultimate healing for that person would be the integration of the personalities or parts, what is more important is that each personality be set free from torment.

This is accomplished by bringing each personality to receive Christ as their Savior and deliver each part from any demonic oppression.

Now as I've mentioned, physical trauma can also lead to spiritual trauma. This, of course, would be the case of a person having an accident which would create a fear of that activity, but just the memory of the incident could bring fear, anxiety, anger, etc. Sometimes the memory of traumatic events is suppressed as a physical protective response. However, the trauma will likely be in the cellular memory and will still need to be dealt with. This can be healed by placing your hand on the person's head and commanding trauma out of the memories of the incident even down to the cellular level.

Since trauma can get down into the cellular level, trauma can also be generational.
That is, the trauma can be passed from one generation to the next. This is best addressed similar to the breaking of generational curses by pleading the blood of Christ over the generational line, removing every right of the demonic to afflict you because of any generational trauma, and removing trauma off the generational line in Jesus name.

I suppose one could use the label of PTSD (post-traumatic stress disorder) for all negative effects from traumatic incidents. When we think of PTSD, we tend to think primarily of the military, but this can refer to many other traumatic events as well. Many times it's not just physical issues that need to be healed related to the physical trauma, but spiritual as well. One particular case comes to mind that we experienced when doing a deliverance. We got a call from a parent for help after her teenage daughter tried to hang herself the night before. We usually like to have people come to us for deliverance, but in times like this we do house calls. That way we can clean the house spiritually as well as minister to the person. As we walked into the bedroom, we tried to get a sense for demonic presence. Either way, we pled the blood of Christ over the room, commanded any demonic sprits to leave, and commanded them not to return. I'll usually ask the Lord to send angels of protection to guard the location as well. Once the room was dealt with, we ministered to the girl. She said that she was told and convinced by a voice in her head to hang herself. When asked how long she had the voices in her head, she responded all of her life. Since she never knew any different, she thought it was normal, and she assumed it was just the two sides of her brain communicating. The Holy Spirit quickly revealed the door to the issue. It turned out that the girl suffered severe trauma during child birth. She actually had her shoulder broken in the process. So, we walked her through forgiveness of all involved. Even though it was not intentional, it's still important to forgive. Then I broke off all of the trauma in Jesus name. What she experienced next is what makes me love this ministry. I commanded all effects of the trauma to be healed and commanded the demonic that came in through that incident to leave in Jesus name. The girl then said she heard a voice say, "You are now free." She said it was a different voice. We knew immediately it was the Holy Spirit. She said she also saw darkness come out from her; it was placed in a box and taken away by two angels. Her mom said days later that she had been glowing ever since.

In each case mentioned above, just like the last one, casting out or off the demonic will be necessary after the trauma and other doors have been dealt with.

Here are prayers to break off trauma and the effects thereof:
- *I command all trauma from _____ (fill in with description of experience) to leave in Jesus name.*
- *I command all trauma out of my memory, even down to the cellular level in Jesus name.*
- *I command all effects of the trauma to be reversed and healed in Jesus name.*

- *I command anything of the enemy that came in through the trauma to leave now and go wherever Jesus tells you to go in Jesus name.*

SPIRITS OF INFIRMITY

A spirit of infirmity or affliction is one that brings physical suffering. Sometimes the affliction may be completely caused from the spirit itself, and sometimes the spirit may create the infirmity. Just as there are healing angels, there are spirits of affliction of different types.

We see a deaf and dumb spirit mentioned in Mark.

> Mark 9:25
> 25 When Jesus saw that the people came running together, He rebuked the unclean spirit, saying to it, "Deaf and dumb spirit, I command you, come out of him and enter him no more!"

There is a spirit of infirmity that kept a lady bent over as noted in Luke.

> Luke 13:10-13
> 10 Now He was teaching in one of the synagogues on the Sabbath. 11 And behold, there was a woman who had a spirit of infirmity eighteen years, and was bent over and could in no

way raise herself up. 12 But when Jesus saw her, He called her to Him and said to her, "Woman, you are loosed from your infirmity." 13 And He laid His hands on her, and immediately she was made straight, and glorified God.

Sometimes the spirit will not be the only problem, but rather be the cause of the problem. It may create a physical problem and be there to reinforce it. In the case of cancer, for example, there is a spirit behind it. That's not to say cancer is not physical. I'm saying that cancer often has a spirit behind it.

Don't get me wrong. I'm not saying there is a demon behind every sickness and infirmity, but in some cases there may be. That is something to be considered when going after the healing with prayer.

One time I was talking to a man I had just met, and while talking to him I got a word of knowledge for pain in his ear. I asked him if by chance he had pain in his ear, and he said that he did. He had it since he got back from Iraq, and the doctors couldn't seem to find the problem. So, I asked if I could pray for him, and he agreed. I prayed that God would heal his ear in Jesus name, and immediately the pain dropped from his ear to his jaw. I did it again out of curiosity because this was kind of new to me at the time, and the pain went to the back of his throat. So, I then commanded that afflicting spirit to leave him in Jesus name, and the pain left. This was an example of an afflicting spirit with no attachment. An interesting thing to note here is that it didn't leave until I took authority over it (commanded it to leave in Jesus name).

When I suspect there is an afflicting spirit causing the infirmity, I'll first just try to command it to go. However, rather than leave, it will sometimes get worse instead. This is an indication that the spirit believes it has a legal right to be there.

When you pray for the sick, four things can happen:

1. Nothing, which is a bummer. We want them to be healed, and this tells us nothing.
2. They get better. Praise God! This is what we want.
3. The pain associated with their infirmity immediately moves. This is not normal, and of course not what we wanted when we prayed.
4. The pain associated with their infirmity immediately gets worse. This is not normal, and of course not what we wanted when we prayed.

This is what I have learned as a rule of thumb. If the pain moves, it's usually an afflicting spirit with no attachment. If the pain gets worse, it's an afflicting spirit with an attachment. By saying the spirit has an attachment, I mean the afflicting sprit believes it has a legal right to be there. When the spirit has no attachment, it can just be commanded off in Jesus name. However, when the spirit has an attachment, it tends to dig in and not let go because it believes it has a right to be there. Again, that is not a law. I've seen exceptions, but that has commonly been my experience.

It's always God's will for us to live healthy in spirit, soul, and body.

> 3 John 2
> Beloved, I pray that you may prosper in all things and be in health, just as your soul prospers.

It is also God's will for us to have victory over the enemy. However, when there is a soul issue that needs to be corrected, victory over an afflicting spirit can't be accomplished until we deal with that soul issue first. I have seen this many times when doing an inner healing or deliverance session. If the deliverance becomes a power encounter only where, by God's authority, I see the evil spirit leave, he will be right back later if the soul issue isn't dealt with.

One common barrier to healing is believing a lie, such as, "I'm not worthy of healing." An example that comes to mind is a young lady who had tendonitis for which we prayed. It got healed, but it came back after only a few days. This happened a few weeks in a row. So, we wondered why the healing wasn't staying. It turned out that she didn't feel worthy of her healing because she had such a low self-image. We broke off the power of that lie and helped her see how God viewed her. She then received healing, and it didn't get stolen.

Another example that comes to mind is one of my favorite healing experiences. Some friends of ours came to us and asked if we would join them to pray for their friend who was suffering from heart failure. He was actually going to be placed into hospice care. One of our friends with us can sometimes see in the spirit. When her husband and I prayed for their friend to have a new heart, she saw an angel show up with a heart in his hand. However, their friend wouldn't receive the new heart. So, we prayed. She then heard the word unworthy. So, we realized that he felt unworthy of receiving the new heart. After walking him through the breaking off of that lie and helping him see things from God's perspective, we prayed again. This time he was able to receive the heart, and his color immediately changed from a pasty white to a healthy color. The next day, he contacted our common friend to say that he had just gone for a swim and was able to swim a mile without any loss of breath. Simply amazing.

Again, anytime you believe a lie of the enemy you empower him. Many times, soul issues could manifest in a form of physical affliction. So, the physical affliction may just be a sign of a much deeper issue. Sometimes when the soul issue is healed, the physical manifestation may just get healed as well. Other times, it may just make way for the physical healing.

When praying for an affliction caused by a spirit of infirmity, you can just command it to go. Here is an example of what to say, out loud.

I command that affliction off of you now in Jesus name.

Remember, you are using your authority to command it to go in Jesus name. You aren't praying.

OUR POSITIONAL AUTHORITY

Satan can't stop us. All he can do is lie to us about who we are and keep us ignorant about that to which we have access. The Bible says that we are seated in heavenly places. This signifies a place of authority. In fact, according to Revelation we are Kings.

> Revelation 1:6
> and **has made us kings** and priests to His God and Father, to Him be glory and dominion forever and ever. Amen.

I'm not saying we should be arrogant about our identity in Christ, but we should have a confidence in who we are. That's important because the enemy will challenge our identity.

Next, know that there is power when we use the name of Jesus. This is because, according to Paul, we are ambassadors for Christ (2 Cor 5:20). We are ambassadors of the Kingdom of God to this earth. As with any ambassador, we carry the authority of the one we represent. In our case we represent the King of Kings, Jesus Christ.

In Luke 10, Jesus sends out seventy disciples to heal the sick and proclaim that the kingdom of God has come near to them. Then when they returned, it says they were full of joy and even a bit surprised at their power over the demonic.

> Luke 10:17-19
> Then the seventy returned with joy, saying, "Lord, even the demons are subject to us in Your name."
> And He said to them, "I saw Satan fall like lightning from heaven.
> Behold, I give you the authority to trample on serpents and scorpions, and over all the power of the enemy, and nothing shall by any means hurt you.

The Lord's name is key. The name of Jesus is very powerful. Know that He gives us the authority to use it as His ambassadors.

In Acts 19 we see a couple of guys trying to use Jesus name to cast out demons, but they had no relationship with Jesus.

> Acts 19:14-16
> Seven sons of Sceva, a Jewish chief priest, were doing this. One day the evil spirit answered them, "Jesus I know, and Paul I know about, but who are you?" Then the man who had the evil spirit jumped on them and overpowered them all. He gave them such a beating that they ran out of the house naked and bleeding.

If ever we were confronted with a demon that asked, "Who are you?", what would we respond? If we just see ourselves as sinners saved by grace, or just a lowly beggar that God has shown mercy, then we don't see ourselves with a proper view. That's not what Jesus would say about us.

In Revelation it says that on Jesus' thigh it's written King of Kings and Lord of Lords. So who are these kings over which He is King? You and I. Our spirits are seated in heavenly places (Eph 2:6). However, our authority still comes in whom we represent. So, we can command the demonic to go in Jesus' name.

As Christians, we need to be confident of our authority for ministering deliverance. As with any responsibility given, one needs the tools and authority to accomplish the job. This is why at the very beginning of the great commission given in Matthew 28, Jesus starts by addressing authority.

> Matthew 28:18-20
> 18 And Jesus came and spoke to them, saying, "**All authority has been given to Me in heaven and on earth.** 19 **Go therefore** and make disciples of all the nations, baptizing them in the name of the Father and of the Son and of the Holy Spirit, 20 teaching them to observe all things that I have commanded you; and lo, I am with you always, even to the end of the age." Amen.

He says all authority has been given to Him in heaven and on earth. This is important to note because prior to the cross Satan had stolen the authority on earth from man, but Jesus reclaimed it. This leaves no authority for Satan anywhere. While he was the prince of the earth and could at one time offer the kingdoms of the world to Jesus, he now has nothing.

So again, as ambassadors of Christ, we are delegated authority to represent Him. There is power associated with this authority. This is why the great commission is preceded with this statement by Jesus, "All authority in heaven and on earth has been given to me." The next words He says are, "Go therefore." So, the fact that Jesus has been given all authority is critical to the ability to carry out the great commission.

As I mentioned in the previous chapter, the power of the anointing plays a role as well. I've had times where I've laid my hand on an affliction and the pain immediately moved because it was an afflicting spirit. If you think that sounds strange, it shouldn't when you realize that according to Acts 19:12 the apostle Paul carried so much anointing of the Holy Spirit that a handkerchief that he touched could bring healing and drive out demons. That's amazing.

The presence of God on a person will vary from time to time, at least for your average believer like me. Thankfully, we also carry authority when needed. What does this authority do for us as His ambassadors? Well, in Luke 10:19 it said that Jesus had given authority to trample on snakes and scorpions and to overcome all the powers of the enemy.

In that verse the snakes and scorpions represent demons and evil spirits. As Jesus says, we are given authority over them to overcome their power. This is very important in understanding deliverance. We have the authority to deliver those afflicted and demonized and break spiritual strongholds in Jesus name. This authority is tied to faith, however. You need to be confident in who you are in Christ. Too often Christians will try to take authority over the enemy only to be laughed at because the enemy knows that person has no real faith in who he is in Christ.

Someone in the Bible who really understood authority was the centurion mentioned in Luke chapter 7. He went to see Jesus because his servant was sick and about to die. He told Jesus, "But say the word, and my servant will be healed." He told Jesus to just say the word because he understood authority and that this could be handled with authority. Jesus was amazed at the level of faith that the centurion had. Likewise, we need to have an understanding and faith in Jesus' authority and then in our authority as His ambassadors. When a Christian states something in Jesus' name, it carries the same type of authority.

The Role of the Anointing Power of the Holy Spirit

Most of the work a police officer does can be done without the use of force. Usually, there is a respect for the authority he carries and that which he represents. Such is also the case for the Christian when it comes to dealing with the demonic. The demonic will usually respond to our authority if we are confident in who we are and who we represent.

However, there are some that need to be reminded of our authority, and even then they may still not respect our authority. This is why, like a soldier or police officer, we have weapons of warfare.

> 2 Corinthians 10:4
> For the weapons of our warfare are not carnal but mighty in God for pulling down strongholds

Our anointing is one of those powerful weapons. There have been times when the demonic would manifest and act out when we are trying to cast them out. I would lay my hand on the person while commanding the demon to stop manifesting, interfering, or leave if it no longer had a legal right to be there. This would be more effective than just commanding it without the laying on of my hand.

I remember one time I had a very stubborn demon that just wouldn't go. I finally just laid my hands on the person and started filling him with the Spirit. As a result, the demon left because it couldn't take tangible anointing of the Holy Spirit.

In Matthew 12:43 it says, "When an unclean spirit goes out of a man, he goes through dry places, seeking rest, and finds none." Why does it go from one dry place to another? Well, the Holy Spirit is often referred to as many wet symbolisms such as a river, as oil, an anointing, a baptism, etc. So, it makes sense they would desire a dry place (such as the dead dry bones) which shows a lack of the Holy Spirit.

The demonic hates the anointing. One time I was filling a young lady who was very demonized with the Holy Spirit by the laying on of my hands in an attempt to push out the demons, and the demons started yelling, "This is so gross" and started pulling her away. Being successful at pushing the demonic out with filling with the Holy Spirit by the laying on of hands doesn't always work, and it's not the best method to get a person free.

To avoid any confusion, I'd like to point out that this is different than the laying on of hands to cast demons out. When laying hands on a person to cast out demons, you are commanding the demons to go. The purpose of the laying on of hands when casting them out is to help enforce the command. However, when they leave due to the laying on of hands to fill/impart the Holy Spirit, it's a side effect.

The most amazing story I have of the demonic leaving while laying on of hands to fill the person with the Holy Spirit was in India. I actually didn't know that was happening at the time. I got the full story from the local pastor who shared with me later. While in India we held an outreach meeting for the youth in the area. A teenage boy was asked by a girl who knew him if he was interested in going. At first he said no, but when she said there was free food and air conditioning, he agreed to attend. I preached the gospel to them, and this boy was one of several that received Christ as his Savior. Later someone else taught about the baptism or filling of the Holy Spirit. When the speaker was finished, we invited all forward to be prayed for to receive the baptism of the Holy Spirit, and that teenage boy got in my line. I laid hands on him to fill him with the Holy Spirit and, unknowingly, was casting out several demons at the same time. The amazing thing was that prior to this event, the boy was known in his neighborhood for running around at night throwing rocks at houses, screaming, and beating people up on the street. He went home completely set free and a new person in Jesus Christ. He got rid of his evil movies and music and started going to church. Several people in the neighborhood asked his mother what happened to him, and she contacted the pastor to tell him about her changed son.

While these stories showed some success of the demonic getting kicked out while filling a person with the Holy Spirit, I don't suggest filling people with the Holy Spirt as a method to kick out the demonic. I'm mostly just sharing this to illustrate the effect of the anointing. Again, the laying of hands on a person to cast out demons is to assist in the commanding of demons to go. It's combining of power and authority. So, I might lay my hands a person while commanding the demons to leave, but my focus in that case is getting rid of the demons, not filling the person with the Holy Spirit.

WARFARE TACTICS AND CALLING ON HEAVENLY REALMS

In case it's not obvious, deliverance is war. You're taking ground back from the enemy. So, as in war, there are good tactics to use when ministering deliverance.

When dealing with very demonized people, there is likely a hierarchy of demonic present. When the demonic have a large stronghold and a lot of history with a place or person, they tend to be more resistant than normal to leaving their location and assignment. I would suggest for these type of cases to cut off the demonic from any communication or support. You could pray and ask Jesus to do that, or just decree that all communication be cut off in Jesus name. Then I would also use my authority to tell the demonic that they can't transfer their assignment in Jesus name.

Another tactic can be learned from the story of Gideon. When he attacked the enemy, the Lord caused confusion in the camp, even to the point where they turned on each other. So, I will sometimes ask the Lord to confuse the enemy.

Lastly, calling for support is helpful. You may think it's automatic to have angelic support, but asking for it really makes a difference. One of the most valuable things I've learned when doing deliverance was to partner with angels. While our prayers can often create angelic action, it can sometimes be very helpful to ask for God to release them to assist us. The angelic are ready to assist, but they respond to direction. That direction primarily comes from God, but we are also seated in heavenly places with Christ. In view of that, angels respond to our words and actions as well, as long as it aligns with God's will.

I first got the revelation of asking for angelic assistance from a dream I had. In the dream I got a call from someone at church to come over because they had a lot of demonic activity in their house. When I arrived, they told me that most of it was in the basement. So, I went down there to investigate. The basement was dimly lit and consisted of a series of rooms on both sides of a hallway. The doors to all of the rooms were closed, but I could hear demonic sounds, cries, and noises behind all of the doors. I then began to feel a little overwhelmed. So, I asked God for some help. I immediately noticed a small table in the hallway with a note on it. It was a note from God, informing me all of the different types of angels He sent to assist me and how many of each type. I then saw a glow behind me, and as I turned around there was an army of angels standing behind me waiting for me to take action. I then simply walked down the hall, and in groups they opened each door and ran in. I could hear fighting going on in each room they entered. They started to get impatient and began running ahead of me to finish off the work. I then woke up and pondered the dream.

Soon after I had that dream, I was reading my Bible during my time with the Lord. I read the passage where Jesus told Peter that He could call upon the Father to release twelve legions of angels to come to His assistance. I then had this thought come to my mind: How many angels could be released to come to my assistance?

As I mentioned earlier, we have access to the kingdom of heaven. Given keys means given access to.

In Matthew 16:19 Jesus says

19 "And **I will give you the keys of the kingdom of heaven**, and whatever you bind on earth will be bound in heaven, and whatever you loose on earth will be loosed in heaven."

This passage talks about our authority to bind and loosen. We have been given authority over all bondage in Jesus name. Whatever we bind (i.e. enemy) or loosen (i.e. those in bondage by the enemy) here on earth, God will reinforce in the heavenly realms to make it a realization here on earth.

An example of a physical manifestation of this is shown in Mark 7:33-35 where a man's ears are opened and his tongue is loosened.

Mark 7:33-35

33 And He took him aside from the multitude, and put His fingers in his ears, and He spat and touched his tongue. 34 Then, looking up to heaven, He sighed, and said to him, "Ephphatha," that is, "Be opened." 35 Immediately his ears were opened, and the impediment of his tongue was loosed, and he spoke plainly.

Keys to the kingdom of heaven are also mentioned in Matthew 16:19. So, we have access to the things in heaven to help us with ministry. This can be for a variety of things, but since we are talking about deliverance I will focus specifically on that purpose. The most obvious to me would be having access to heaven's angelic army.

So, I started being more intentional about using or partnering with angels. We can ask Jesus to release angels to help. We have angels assigned to us for ministry. However, when needed in a particular

75

situation, Jesus can release even more angels than we normally have assisting us when we ask Him.

After a difficult but successful deliverance, one that had very many strong and violent demons, I noticed myself shaking the next day. I had PTSD that I needed to break off of myself. So, I told God I quit and to stop sending those needing deliverance to me. I then felt bad, and I sensed the Holy Spirit say, "Then who should I send them to?" Obviously, there are others that He could send them to, but I did know that He called me to this ministry. So I immediately repented. However, I said, "I'll do this ministry on two conditions. First, I want your manifest presence here with me when it's a difficult situation, and I'll want your assistance. Second, I want an angelic upgrade."

The Lord provides what we need for ministry, but sometimes we need to ask for it.

> John 14:13-14
> 13 And whatever you ask in My name, that I will do, that the Father may be glorified in the Son. 14 If you ask anything in My name, I will do it.

In this case, He answered right away. The very next day we had another very rebellious demon that manifested by saying no in a deep eerie voice and started clawing the table when I tried to lead a young lady in a prayer of rededication to Christ. I asked the Lord to make this demon obey since he was being rebellious. The demon made this smirk look through the girl, trying to imply it's doing no good. I kept asking the Lord to turn up the heat on him until the smile left. I then called upon the angelic for help to bind the demon and place him in a closet so he would not interfere. Things then went very smoothly without the interference of the demonic. Once I dealt with the issues that the Holy Spirit revealed, I then had the demons sent away since they no longer had any legal right to be there.

I had two people in the room that could see in the spirit realm during the deliverance session, and when we were done, I asked them what they saw. To my surprise, they both said they saw a cloud. They said it was a good cloud that looked like it was full of gold dust. To me that was an indication that the Lord was there in our presence providing assistance.

I had other sessions where the demonic were rebellious and even a bit violent. When I asked for the angelic host to be released and to come assist, a look of terror came on the face of the one that was manifesting the demon. The person looked up in all directions. At first, I thought they were seeing the angels coming. It then occurred to me they were looking up because the angels were so large.

Some demons like to scream through the person as a manifestation. This can be unnerving for those around, as well as annoying. So, what I'll often do in this case is ask the angelic to bind and gag the demonic. Also, when the demons are getting kicked out, I'll command them to go quietly. If they still start to manifest on the way out, I'll ask the angelic to enforce that they go quietly. You can ask the Lord to send assistance to make them go quietly as well.

THIS TYPE ONLY COMES OUT BY PRAYER AND FASTING

Deliverance is entering into spiritual battle, and the enemy doesn't like to be kicked out. So, be prepared. First, we need to be healthy. Prepare yourself daily. Just as your physical strength is dependent on regular nourishment and rest, so is the case with your spirit man. We need our rest, and we need to feed our minds and spirits with spiritual nourishment from God's Word and time in His presence. Whatever ushers you into the presence of God is key to your success. It might be time in His Word. It might be a time of praying in the Spirit. It may be time in vibrant praise. It may be time soaking in meditation, worship, and just being aware of Him. These are daily types of activities. There are also practices that we should do on occasion to strengthen us even further, such as fasting.

An example of this can be seen in Judges 20 when the Israelites go to fight the Benjamites. There were two times that Israel asked God if they should go fight the Benjamites, and God said yes. Yet, both times they were defeated. In fact, they lost thousands of men. They asked God, and God said yes. So, it was God's will for them to fight, yet they lost both times. See even though they asked God if they should go, they went without proper preparation. Then they asked a third time, and again God said yes. However, this time they fasted and offered burnt sacrifices, and when they went out, they had victory. They asked each time, but it wasn't until they did their own preparation through sacrifices and offerings that they had the victory.

Likewise, when the disciples couldn't cast the demon out of the boy in Mark 9, they asked Jesus why they failed.

> Mark 9:28-29
> 28 And when He had come into the house, His disciples asked Him privately, "Why could we not cast it out?"
> 29 So He said to them, **"This kind can come out by nothing but prayer and fasting."**

This kind you will only defeat after you properly prepare yourselves spiritually. It's not that you fast to get rid of the demon. You fast to prepare yourself for when you are faced with a demon of that kind.

So, what provision or strengthening did they need to fast in order to prepare for encountering a demon of that type? Surprisingly it wasn't anointing (I think that is very helpful as well). It was faith. You find this in the parallel account in Matthew 17.

> Matthew 17:19-21
> 19 Then the disciples came to Jesus privately and said, "Why could we not cast it out?" 20 So Jesus said to them, **"Because of your unbelief**; for assuredly, I say to you, if you have **faith as a mustard seed**, you will say to this mountain, 'Move from here to there,' and it will move; and nothing will be impossible for you. 21 However, this kind does not go out except by prayer and fasting."

One might ask the question: Didn't they have a mustard seed of faith? After all, they attempted to cast it out, and they had success with casting out other demons. In fact, they were surprised that they couldn't cast this one out. Let me start by saying that unbelief mentioned in verse 20 could be translated little faith. To distinguish this from a mustard seed of faith (also little), it may not be quantity or size, as much as referring to a lasting faith (duration). I understood this because I've experienced similar situations. The thing about this "type" of demon is that it's violent. The thing that surprises me when I read this story in Mark's account is that the demon didn't leave quietly. It cried out and convulsed the boy on the way out. I'm surprised because this is Jesus doing the deliverance. So, this "type" of demon is the very rebellious and violent type. The thing about this type of demon is they will try to shake your faith. This is why some try to put on a show by all kinds of strange manifestations, such as slither like a snake, roll their eyes back into their head, or talk in a strange voice. I've even had one demon smirk at me when I asked Jesus for help and asked Jesus to put pressure on the demon. The demon tried to show that it wasn't doing any good. So, I calmly waited a minute, and the demon started to squirm in discomfort. Those types of demons try to intimidate and make you question your power and authority. I've even had a demon tell me I had no authority. To which I quickly reminded him that I do because of who I am in Christ. So, the prayer and fasting is to strengthen ourselves so that our faith can't be shaken.

Those like me, who can't see angels with their natural eyes, need to take by faith what's present to assist you. Even if you have mighty angels there to assist, you are still in charge. The angelic isn't going to take action without you asserting your authority in the situation. So, if the enemy can get you to lose faith, he's won the battle.

THE DEMONIC ARE POSSESSIVE AND TERRITORIAL

The demonic would love to inhabit people, but they can attach themselves to objects and locations as well. I've heard stories of missionaries that have a hard time destroying idols until they pray over them. As you would expect, if you have an idol in your house, there may be demonic activity that is invited in because of it. Sometimes though the object that invites the demonic in may not be so obvious. As I mentioned previously, I felt the demonic crawl on me when I handled a Ouija board. Sometime when the occult is in a family for a while, they may look at things like a Ouija board just as a relic and keep it as an heirloom. What they don't realize is that there are demonic attachments to it and will cause all kinds of problems for that house, especially in the room it is kept in. I've been to a few houses that some would say are haunted. Objects may float or a room is unexplainably cold. One house we were asked to go to had vampire paintings in it because they thought it was cool. What they didn't know was that it was a source for the demonic to be in their home. This doesn't just cause strange manifestations that may lead to the house seeming to be haunted, but will usually create problems for the family, especially severe sickness.

Once the demonic get assigned or invited into a place, they don't like to leave. That is why some may think they see the spirits or ghosts of grandparents. The demonic have gotten so familiar with those people they mimic the person once they are deceased. Their desire to stay at a location can be seen when Jesus is about to cast out legion from the demoniac. Legion asked that they wouldn't be sent out of the country.

> Mark 5:9-10
> 9 Then He asked him, "What is your name?"
> And he answered, saying, "My name is Legion; for we are many." 10 Also **he begged Him earnestly that He would not send them out of the country.**

They also love to possess something. So, they asked to be sent into nearby pigs.

> Mark 5:11-12
> 11 Now a large herd of swine was feeding there near the mountains. 12 So all the demons begged Him, saying, "**Send us to the swine, that we may enter them.**"

As a result, we see the pigs are so miserable they immediately go kill themselves.

It doesn't need to be occult type of activity that invite the demonic into a location. One house that I was asked to go to had a lot of demonic activity. It turned out that the previous owner was deep into pornography. A notebook was found that he used to journal his activity. One might not think of just sinful habits creating an environment that welcomes the demonic, but it does. We love to have physically secure houses, but too many unknowingly open up pathways in their home for the demonic with their hidden sin. Harmless sin is an oxymoron. We all need to seek to create a safe home spiritually just as much, if not even more, than physically. That being said, you can ask for angels of protection to be released to you for your home. I've had a seer (someone who sees in the spirit realm with their natural eyes) tell me that I have two large armed angels standing guard at the front door of my house.

Having a Home Court Advantage – Creating an Environment of Worship

Sometimes we get invited to speak at churches. At one particular church, over lunch a pastor asked me where we do our freedom sessions. To his surprise we said that we like to do them out of our home. I told him it's like having a home court advantage. We have a sign on our front door that says, "In this house we serve the Lord. Don't be surprised if you feel His presence." Creating an atmosphere that hosts God's presence is very powerful and helpful.

When we enter into worship, it not only affects us, it affects our whole environment, including those around us. Remember Paul and Silas in Acts 16? They were in jail and chained. What did they do? They prayed, but then what? They sang praises. When they did that, the Bible says an earthquake occurred. Doors opened, and chains broke. This is literally physical in this story, but the same holds true in the spiritual as well. Praise opens spiritual doors; praise breaks spiritual chains and spiritual bonds. Doors opening and chains breaking is a picture of evangelism and deliverance. Doors or hearts are open. Chains of sin are broken. Praise is powerful!

Now in the story of Paul and Silas in jail, the earthquake happens, and it makes sense that it could have opened the doors. However, chains were loosed, and that doesn't occur from an earthquake. What is my point? In the story it wasn't just Paul's and Silas's chains that opened, but everyone's. Their praise had an effect on their whole environment, and that wasn't just an accident. And what was the result of it all? People got saved! So, it's a picture of how we create an atmosphere for those to come into the kingdom.

There is power in the presence of God, or one could say the presence of God is what brings power. This is something that can't be easily explained until you have experienced it. We tend to think God is everywhere. While that is theologically possible, it's at minimum abstract. When I say God is more present in one place than another, that may seem abstract as well, but it's tangible too. In a dream Jacob saw angels ascending and descending, and he said, "God is in this place." Even though this was in a dream, the presence of God was tangible. He saw it, and he heard God. There are times when you can feel the presence of evil. It's tangible. Likewise, there are times you can feel a strong presence of God. It's tangible, and it's awesome.

In those places and times when I have been in the strong presence of God, my spiritual gifts are greatly magnified. So, what does this mean? Simple, with the presence of God comes power. Because there is power in the presence of God, it also empowers my gifts, such as my gift of healing. It's like the gifts are power tools, but without being hooked up to the power source, they can't do anything.

My wife and I used to head up a healing ministry, and we had a place called a healing room where people could come for prayer. One night we experienced a healing momentum in our ministry where the presence of God became so strong a couple of people got healed just by walking through the door of the healing room.

85

It's similar with deliverance. Besides prayer, worship is probably the most underestimated power in this world. In the spiritual realm, worship is like an act of violence. It's powerful. A friend of mine told me a story of a guy calling his church because his wife was manifesting a demon. The pastor called my friend for help, and together they tried laboriously to cast out the demon. They did everything to command this demon to go, but it wouldn't. So, they decided to worship. As they stood there and sang praises to God, the demon couldn't handle it, and it left. A great peace came over the woman, and she ended up giving her life to the Lord.

As I look at the life of David, who was described in the Bible as a man after God's own heart, I also see that he was a mighty warrior. To be a mighty warrior, you need to have courage. David's source of courage was his relationship with the Lord. And that relationship was forged out of worship and meditation on God's Word. David was a worshiper. He worshiped God with his harp. He wrote psalms of praise to the Lord. We see David referred to as Israel's singer of songs in 2 Samuel 23:1, and in 2 Samuel 6 we see David dancing before the Lord with all his might. Worship is a key to being a warrior.

If someone has a stressful home environment, I challenge them to have everyone in the house listen to nothing but Christian praise and worship music for a whole day. These days, there is such a wide variety of Christian music that you will find something for everyone's taste. They will see a difference at the end of that day. The reason they will see a difference is that Christian praise and worship music influences behavior. In the verses above Paul contrasts being drunk with wine with being filled with the Spirit. The reason is that he's using an analogy to point out how the Holy Spirit will have influence on our behavior. As we fill ourselves with more of Him, the fruit of the Spirit becomes more evident.

As I said earlier, praise and worship affects the environment. It attracts the glory of God (His manifest presence). The thing about the manifest presence of God is that while it makes things easier, the demonic hate it. So, those being oppressed might not even be able to come into the house, and if they do, they might start manifesting right away. It's still worth it though because most of the time they will still come in, and the session will go much faster and easier as the presence of God exposes the demonic and helps bring the freedom.

Ministering Over Distance

Doing deliverance over long distance may seem like something that might not normally be considered, but in this age of technology it's very possible. I've held freedom sessions (what we call our deliverance ministry) over Skype and over video services as well. It's not as ideal as being there, but I found that it worked very well.

There is even more that can be done remotely in the spirit realm. An example of ministering remotely can be found in Matthew 15:22-28. In this passage a woman of Canaan came to see Jesus because her daughter was severely demon-possessed. After a bit of a discussion, Jesus answered and said to her, "O woman, great is your faith! Let it be to you as you desire." And her daughter was healed from that very hour. I've read that several times, and there's a lot to gleam from this interesting passage. One day a thought hit me. Jesus did a deliverance on her daughter without being there and with no interaction with the daughter. I pondered this and thought about the reasons we tend to need interaction with the person we are helping. I came up with two possible reasons.

The first reason that it's often helpful to interact in person is to determine if they want to be free. This may seem like a silly reason because you may think wouldn't everyone want to be free. Surprisingly, the answer is no. Some would rather keep their lifestyle or may have some other reason. The point is there are some that don't want help. We especially have encountered this with parents with troubled teens. We tell them that we can't help if the teen doesn't want help. Usually they do want help, but not always. That's why in John 5 Jesus asks the man by the Pool of Bethesda if he would want to be healed. This seems like a ridiculous question, but we need to know. Some people just get comfortable in their circumstance, and they often agree with the lie that it will never change.

The second reason is that if there is a stronghold it's easier to identify. This is especially true if they need to renounce something that they personally had done that opened a door to the demonic.

Now let me say there are cases where neither one of these situations exists. That is the person needing freedom wants it, and they are not able for some reason to meet, not even with technology. It's a rare case, but they exist. For example, we have had cases where a teen is brought to our house and he wants freedom, but the demonic changes his mind about coming inside when he arrives. We could still do some limited amount of ministry. The authority that the Lord has given us has no limits to distance.

Other situations may tend to be more for spiritual warfare than deliverance, but it's related. For example, one time a lady at my church needed freedom from oppression. After leading her in a quick session that brought freedom, it was brought to our attention that her apartment had an oppressive darkness around it. So, I asked the Lord to release the angelic to spiritually cleanse her apartment and assign some to stand guard there. I also asked that the Lord release His presence in her apartment. The lady returned the next week saying that things had been very different since I did that.

Then there is the case where the physical isn't involved in the deliverance at all. Our spirit isn't limited by our bodies. One deliverance session that was a little more involved became tiring, and we needed to end it before we were done. That is unusual, but in some cases necessary. That night I continued to do deliverance in my sleep. The person being ministered to also dreamt that I was doing deliverance on them. When they woke up, they felt more freedom. There is no doubt in my mind that my spirit continued what was started in the physical.

Ministry Etiquette

You want to create an environment where those ministered to feel safe and cared for. They need to know that they can trust you and that they won't feel judged. For example, if they share activities with you that are very sick, perverted, or shocking in which they have participated, you need to keep a straight face. Be sure to keep things confidential. In fact, it's a good idea to throw notes away right after the session is done. At the same time if they share experiences that were very hurtful, you should always act with compassion. That is to be our motivation. Make sure the person feels cared for and loved. They are the priority.

Never minister alone. In this day of so much false accusation, it's a good idea to have witnesses and accountability. At least one of the people ministering should be of the same sex as the person being ministered to, and any of the opposite sex should offer to step out of the room when dealing with sexual topics. It's also good to be able to hand off the process if you need to take a break. That being said, it's good to have only one person minister at a time. It keeps things from being diverted off track, and it shows a clear line of authority to the demonic. If one has a revelation or idea, they should quietly let the leader know. He can then address it when he feels appropriate. Also, keep the number present to a minimum. Otherwise, it can be intimidating and distracting. I would suggest not more than three people in total (not including those coming for ministry) be involved in the deliverance process. Anyone sitting in should be cleared with the person receiving ministry. If they are not part of the few ministering, they should stay quiet and intercede in prayer. It is good to have others not present intercede as well.

If there is strong manifestation, stay calm. This will help the person stay calm, and it won't show any weakness to the enemy. The enemy will recognize fear and a lack of confidence. Along with that, don't get in the flesh. For example, don't yell. The demonic can hear fine. Simply talk with authority. Make sure the person being ministered to understands that you are not talking to them, but to the enemy. Explain to the person being ministered to what is happening and help bring them hope and confidence during the session.

It's not a good idea to minister in public to those manifesting the demonic. This can be embarrassing to the person. However, if there is a need for deliverance that comes up in public that won't likely create a scene, it's ok to minister on the spot if this is more convenient than setting up an appointment. For example, I was with some friends at a bar and grill for dinner one time when we prayed for a lady. She was a waitress working there, and she was highlighted to me, even though she wasn't our waitress. It started out that I just prophesied over her tattoos. I then got a word of knowledge for her elbow, prayed for it, and her elbow got healed. Then a lady with us got a word of knowledge for alcoholism. She admitted it was a struggle. In fact, it was creating deep depression within her. She said that she woke up that morning feeling hopeless. We continued to minister, and the waitress received Christ as her Savior. The transformation on her face was amazing. We had no idea it would turn into a little deliverance session and her receiving Christ as her Savior, but God knew.

For some it's hard for them to accept that God really cares about them. They feel their choices have led them to where they are, and they deserve the life they are living. What they don't realize is that Jesus came to give life and life abundantly. Sometimes God can reinforce what He wants to do through a healing. So, we need to keep listening to the Holy Spirit. He might want to do things in a different order than you are planning.

One lady who was suicidal got saved, healed, and delivered. I got a word of knowledge for her elbow, which suffered trauma from abuse. She was shocked that it got completely healed when I prayed for it. It helped reinforce to her that God really cares.

One more thing, when you are going to pray for someone, make sure you ask before you place your hand on them. Be sure to place it only in appropriate places after receiving permission.

WRAPPING UP AND FOLLOW UP STEPS

I've already discussed the importance of making sure the person needing deliverance is saved. Once free, Godly structures need to be put into place where the enemy's strongholds existed. To help start this process, when you come to the end of a deliverance session, the person should also be filled with the Holy Spirit. I'll simply lay my hands on them and ask the Holy Spirit to fill them up, and for His fruit to manifest in their lives. It's also good to coach them on building their spirit up in the area that was weak. This can be done by providing them with declarations of truth to state regularly and scriptures pertinent to their previous stronghold for them to meditate on.

Next, you need to dust off. What I mean by that is to command anything lingering that was released to go where Jesus tells it to go. Also, pray against anything following the person ministered to back to their home. Pray protection against any retaliation against you or your family.

Follow up in a few days to see how the person ministered to is doing. Encourage them that they can stay free without having to do a lot of battle. Reiterate to them about their new identity in Christ and how their identity is based on what Christ has done for us that has given us new life. Remind them of their authority in their identity in Christ. Review some declarations together and pray with them for fresh strength. Encourage them to ask for fresh grace every day first thing in the morning and to expect great things. Remind them to regularly review any encouraging words or pictures the Holy Spirit brought to light, as well as any pertinent verses to meditate on.

Another session may be needed if something was missed or just went hiding. Always ask the Holy Spirit for revelation, but in some cases a questionnaire form might be useful to cover things that you wouldn't normally think of or feel comfortable asking about (such as certain sexual practices).

I hope that you gleamed a lot from this book, and it's my prayer now that you walk in freedom as God intended and help others to do so as well. May God anoint you with dunamis power and equip you to minister to others according to your faith and calling in Jesus name!

About the Author

Steve Dominguez is an author and speaker who has trained others in living out the Christian life in power and authority. He and his wife, Risa, have both served in a variety of ministries including evangelism, healing, and deliverance. Steve has also followed in his father's footsteps in jail ministry for over 35 years.